TRANSING OUR CHILDREN

By Erin Brewer, PhD
with Maria Keffler, MS Ed

Transing Our Children
Erin Brewer, PhD and Maria Keffler, MS Ed

Copyright © 2021, Advocates Protecting Children
ISBN: 9798465402224

Advocates Protecting Children
P.O. Box 41981
Arlington VA, 22204
https://www.advocatesprotectingchildren.org

PRAISE FOR TRANSING OUR CHILDREN

Erin and Maria have hit it out of the park with *Transing Our Children*! We're in a critical era wherein children are being relentlessly indoctrinated with the false ideology that transgenderism is a catch-all reason for their problems and transition is the cure-all solution. Likewise, parents are emotionally blackmailed that the choice is transition of their child or suicide. Neither sales pitch is true. Erin and Maria have put together a remarkably thorough, yet concise and highly readable, book guiding the reader through what they need to know to address the component issues and the movement. A great resource for protecting our children!

—Andre Van Mol, MD
Board-certified family physician;
Co-chair, Committee on Adolescent Sexuality,
American College of Pediatricians;
Co-chair, Sexual and Gender Identity Task Force,
Christian Medical & Dental Association

Erin Brewer and Maria Keffler have created a compact and powerful resource for anyone seeking straightforward, evidence-based answers to the confusing onslaught of ideological messaging surrounding the transgender phenomenon. They offer readers well-documented factual vignettes explaining the hot button issues grabbing headlines and infiltrating our social institutions, including medicalization of our children, the suicide extortion being foisted on parents, the harms of medical transitioning and the vilification of detransitioners.

Interspersed with the evidence-based factual discussions are personal stories of those who were swept into and harmed by the transgender agenda. These stories are emotional and heartfelt, showing the human cost of this phenomenon.

Transing Our Children is an invaluable resource for those who want to understand the phenomenon without having to delve into reams of medical studies and scientific white papers. It will empower readers with the knowledge necessary to effectively engage with those who are promoting the agenda and those struggling with its effects.

It is a resource we will be recommending to our clients.

—Mary E. McAlister, Esq.
Child & Parental Rights Campaign
www.childparentrights.org

In 1967 when I was only 12 years old, I thought I was meant to be a boy instead of feeling like something of a "non-girl," as a neighbor stated to my mother to describe me. I discovered Christine Jorgensen's autobiography and the line he wrote, "Nature made a mistake, which I have corrected," and I thought I'd found the answer to my internalized hatred of my female body and the fact that I adored and wanted to marry a woman when I grew up. From that point on until I was in my early thirties, I thought I'd be on the path to having medicine and surgeries to 'correct' the 'otherness' I felt.

I did not understand that my struggles were not about my body or sexual orientation, but the greater flaw of a society that constantly was telegraphing that it would never accept me as I naturally was.

If I were 12 years old today, I definitely would have gone the route of ingesting dangerous puberty blockers and wrong sex hormones, and subjecting my body to life-altering surgeries to transform my secondary sex characteristics to see if I could pass as a male. I thought my job prospects would be better, people would actually listen to my concerns, and that a woman would find me a suitable romantic partner for what could now be accepted as a legal marriage.

Transing Our Children does a fantastic job of injecting a deeply personal vulnerability to the subject of bodily agency along with sexual expression and sexual orientation. It crosses over into territory that involves historical recognition of clinical studies as well as cultural trends while debunking some dangerous narratives being forced upon us all. It also explains why so many of the current mantras being employed to accept the lie of "transgenderism" are based on entities whose main interests involve advancing their own financial security.

As an activist who's interested in abolishing the practice of performing what appears to be likely the largest medical scandal of this century, this book should be on every shelf in every public library as a resource to help parents and citizens in general understand what we are all up against: nothing but a dangerous ideology that functions to undermine and unmoor us from our sexed bodies. If one more 12-year-old girl or boy is only encouraged to believe that they can be any "identity" they want, *Transing Our Children* can be the anecdote for explaining why that concept is really nothing but a solid lie, and how thinking critically can be a lifesaver for our children.

—joey brite
Organizer of nationwide protests
against the transing of children and youth

Transing Our Children addresses this issue with compassion using easy to understand language. A must read for parents, educators, therapists, doctors and legislators. Our situation might be totally different had this book been available when our family was unwillingly dragged into this ideology. Definitely worth sharing with anyone who cares about children.

—Anonymous mother of child
who identifies as transgender

Erin Brewer and Maria Keffler have provided a priceless resource for professionals, parents and their children. We live in Orwellian times. This book will save lives.

—Michelle Cretella, MD
Executive Director,
American College of Pediatricians

Erin Brewer has put together a very useful treatise, *Transing Our Children*, using a series of essays on the various complex aspects of gender incongruence and the proposed therapies so aggressively pushed by the LGBT [sic] activist community. Each session has a specific theme, but as you read through all the sections, you quickly see how they all intertwine. This very effectively serves to reinforce the story she tells. She bravely includes her own personal story as well as those of other victims of the transgender "industry." This is a great reference to share with families and patents who struggle with the innate angst of gender incongruence.

—Dr. Quentin Van Meter
Pediatric Endocrinologist

TABLE OF CONTENTS

ACKNOWLEDGMENTS

A number of quotes were taken from comments on YouTube videos and other places. Transgender-rights activists bully and harass people who speak out against transgender ideology, therefore these comments will be noted with an asterisk, rather than a citation, to protect the privacy and safety of those quoted.

We also want to thank all of those who are tirelessly fighting to save our children and families, risking livelihood, family, and friendships. For safety/privacy reasons, we will not name individuals here, although a number of you are listed in the endnotes for your publicly written and recorded contributions to this fight. For the many who are not public, please know that you are seen, you are appreciated, and you are invaluable.

DEDICATION

To the 7 Sisters and all the victims of the gender industry, especially detransitioners and desisters who are bravely sharing their stories.

FOREWORD

While mapping the recent explosion of gender clinics as the GenderMapper, both in the United States and internationally, I have uncovered ample and incontestable evidence of the gender industry's stranglehold on the narrative about gender dysphoria. The gender industry, which predates on children and mutilates youth and adults alike, is bankrupt to its absolute core. The gender industry cannot be regulated; it must be abolished. This is the mission to which I hold, and it is the mission that Erin Brewer and Maria Keffler hold to as well.

Transing Our Children is the fruit of a deep, wide, and horror-inducing investigation into the twisted world of childhood transgenderism. Brewer and Keffler have applied their analytic and critical-thinking skills to unmask this beast of an ideology, producing this thorough and ground-breaking book.

From the moment I read *The Transexual Empire* by Janice Raymond, I well understood that gender ideology is a tragic disaster for the rights and protections of women and children. As early as 1979 Raymond professed that child "sex role control centers" were already in development. We know that today there are more than 300 child gender clinics and pediatric gender surgeons across North America, and that this booming industry grows by the day.

Transing Our Children is a perfectly timed, critical exposé of the nefarious gender industry and its effects on children, families, and society. This subject is not for the faint-hearted. I expect *Transing Our Children* to be hailed as one of the pivotal analyses in what has become the medical scandal of the 21st century.

—Alix Aharon
Co-founder and board member
of Partners for Ethical Care

INTRODUCTION

"I'm a profoundly unhappy male with unresolved childhood traumas who transitioned as a way to escape myself and I did believe I'm trans but I'm probably just a very effeminate looking/acting guy. Have little to do with the community because I'm attacked for not being supportive of transition, for having doubts, for having thought crimes."

—Posted by ICQME*

"It's heartbreaking. I feel like I'm surrounded by a vast cult of child abuse and medicalized self-harm that's brainwashing youth who are LGB, mentally ill, traumatized, or just insecure. And everyone who speaks out is labeled a bigot! More and more, I feel like I have to do something to stop this madness. If I could save even one kid, it would be worth losing everything."

—Posted by QueenlyFlux*

In a recent study out of Australia, clinicians found that children who receive transgender interventions "appeared to believe that their distress would be completely alleviated if they pursued the pathway of medical treatment." This myth is perpetuated by activists who insist that so-called "affirmative care" (which means "transing kids"), is the only way to address any discomfort a child feels as a result of gender dysphoria.

The Australian study further points out that the "evidence base for all aspects of treatment was and remains sparse."[1]

In other words, children are being given harmful experimental medical interventions despite the existence of little evidence in support of these interventions.

These kids are being denied the opportunity to learn how to manage difficult feelings. Instead, they are being transed.

* * *

Gender dysphoria is a psychiatric diagnosis. First called *gender identity disorder*, now renamed *gender dysphoria*, the term refers to a person whose biological sex doesn't match his or her inner sense of self.

In other words, gender dysphoria describes a disconnect between body and brain.

Those who suffer from gender dysphoria feel that their anxiety and distress is caused by their bodies being the wrong biological sex. Much like patients with obsessive-compulsive disorder incessantly wash their hands, believing that the act of washing will alleviate their distressed feelings, those with gender dysphoria believe that being a different sex than that which they were born will calm their distress. However, even after attempting to transition sexes, the feeling of distress is rarely, if ever, eliminated.

Gender dysphoria is a complicated disorder, and a myriad of factors play into how intensely it may be experienced. Like obsessive-compulsive disorder, the symptoms of gender dysphoria can be managed or resolved. Appropriate treatment for someone with obsessive-compulsive disorder is not to remind the patient of his urge to wash his hands, or to encourage him to wash his hands, or to tell him that it is normal to want to wash his hands so often; rather therapists help people suffering from obsessive-compulsive disorder to manage their compulsion to wash their hands, so that their hands do not become raw and enflamed and susceptible to infection.

In the same way, encouraging someone with gender dysphoria to attempt to transition sexes fails to actually treat the cause of the dysphoria. Like excessive hand washing, transitioning—especially transitioning medically—leads to negative consequences. Some of these consequences—like permanent changes to appearance—are well-known. Many consequences are likely still unknown, because children, teens, and young adults who have medically transitioned have never been tracked over a lifetime to observe and catalog potential side effects.

As a child, I hated my female body. I believed that all the problems I experienced, such as the bullying I suffered and my difficulties fitting in with others, would be fixed if I could just be a boy.

I would put duct tape over my vagina to hide it. Occasionally I would go into a rage and pound my vagina with a rock until I was swollen with bruises. Sometimes, when I brushed my hair, I would experience such self-loathing that I would beat my head with the brush. The sharp bristles tore into my scalp until my hair was matted with blood.

These are not normal behaviors.

The only time other children interacted with me was to tease or taunt me. Packs of girls would corral me in the hallway and force me into the boy's bathroom while they made fun of me. Boys would push me, slap me, and kick me if I came too close to them. I used to carry a great deal of bitterness in my heart towards my schoolmates, but I don't anymore. Now I realize they were responding to me with confusion and fear because I was so different.

This was long before transgenderism was part of our culture.

Thankfully, my school psychologist's recommendation was that teachers and other adults help me accept and appreciate myself as a female. At the time, it wasn't even conceivable that I might be encourage to transition. In fact, the caring adults around me gently nudged me away from my attempts to socially transition by wearing boyish clothes and cutting my hair in a masculine style.

I am thankful that I had supportive teachers and counselors who guided my obsessive focus on my body outward towards more healthy activities. The therapists who taught me how to challenge my internal monologue of constant criticism saved my life. I will be forever grateful for therapists who helped me understand that my gender dysphoria was a coping mechanism that my creative mind came up with to help me make sense of my trauma. I owe a huge debt of gratitude to all the people who helped me realize that it is perfectly okay for a female to express herself in non-stereotypical ways.

But if I were a child today, instead of getting the appropriate help which I needed, I would have been transed.

* * *

Gender dysphoria can have many causes, such as trauma, autism, a misunderstanding about gender non-conformity, and subtle messages children pick up from adults or other children. People who experience gender dysphoria so profoundly into adulthood that they live as the opposite sex have always existed, but until very recently this was extremely rare. Historically, about .003% of the population suffered from gender dysphoria.

The American Psychiatric Associations Diagnostic and Statistical Manual, 5th Edition, (DSM-5), published in 2013, estimates that about 0.005% to 0.014% of males and 0.002% to 0.003% females have gender dysphoria.

However, news reports, anecdotal stories, and surveys suggest that what is now called *transgenderism* is exploding in children and young adults.[2] A jump in numbers this profound may suggest that many of those who today identify as transgender have adopted this identity as a coping mechanism to handle underlying mental health issues.

The emergence of this burgeoning cohort is a direct result of the gender industry's insistence that only one treatment path exists for any child who is gender non-conforming: anyone who suffers from even the slightest twinge of gender dysphoria is put immediately on a path of medicalization via so-called "Affirmative Care."

* * *

Activists call it "affirmation" but this "treatment plan" is nothing less than transing vulnerable children.

Even the World Professional Association for Transgender Health (WPATH), a pro-trans medical advocacy group that set the worldwide standard of care for those with gender dysphoria, admits that gender dysphoria in childhood does not inevitably continue into adulthood, and only six to twenty-three percent of boys and twelve to twenty-seven percent of girls treated in gender clinics showed persistence of their gender dysphoria into adulthood.[3]

That means that up to 94% of boys and 88% of girls desist in having gender dysphoria in adulthood.[4]

As a result of the affirmation model of care, it means that 94% of boys and 88% of girls are being unnecessarily transed. These children are getting the wrong treatment.

Rather than acknowledging that gender dysphoria is often resolved or managed with therapy, transgender-rights activists and their allies in the gender industry actively promote the idea that the only appropriate treatment for gender dysphoria is "transition," which means altering one's external appearance in a way that doesn't match that person's birth sex.

Transing starts with allowing a child or teen to adopt exaggerated, stereotypical behaviors and dress representative of the opposite sex. As the child nears puberty, as young as eight years old, parents are counseled to give their child puberty blockers, which halt a child's normal physical and mental maturation.

After a child has been on puberty blockers for a few years, parents are next led to give their child cross-sex hormones, such as testosterone for girls and estrogen for boys. These hormones force a child's body to develop physical characteristics of the opposite sex. Teens are frequently prescribed cross-sex hormones after just one appointment at a gender clinic.[5]

Gender-confused girls as young as thirteen have radical mastectomies to remove their breasts. Both boys and girls as young as sixteen have surgery to alter their genitals.

No evidence exists to support these transing interventions. No proof shows that they are effective long-term treatments for gender dysphoria.

In fact, these are not "life-saving" medical treatments, as transgender rights activists claim; these dangerous and expensive medical interventions fail to even address the underlying issues causing the child's distress.

Why has this treatment pathway for gender dysphoria been so readily accepted? Because transgender-rights activists have systematically worked to discredit all other treatment methods.

They call anyone who doesn't agree to a child's gender transition "transphobic."

They vilify parents who don't allow a gender-dysphoric children to change their names, use preferred pronouns, or transition sexes. Transgender-rights activists even call these parents abusive.

Transing a child, activists say, is the only way to preventing children from killing themselves.

But if transing really lowered the risk of suicide, then we would see an overall decrease in the rate of suicide as more children are transed. But instead the overall rate of suicide for children and teens has gone up right along with the increase in transing kids, while trans-rights activists go on making their wild, unsubstantiated, and antithetical claims.[6]

* * *

Transgender-rights activists call any therapy that doesn't affirm a child's gender dysphoria "conversion therapy" and are actively working to enact legislation world-wide requiring therapists to affirm a child's identity rather than treat the child for gender dysphoria.

Any who question this narrative or speak out to the contrary are vilified and bullied.

When I first raised concerns about what was happening to children, the following message arrived in my inbox: "You best be getting the f--- out of my town with that transphobic bull---t. You are contributing to our g-d d-mn genocide with how you mock and degrade trans kids."

This was written by a young man my son's age, whom I had watched grow up. We lived in the same apartment complex when he was in elementary school. According to family members, he is autistic and began claiming a trans identity as a result of his struggle to cope with adulthood.

Those who speak publicly about their concerns for how kids are being transed regularly receive harassing messages and threats of violence.

Dr. Kenneth Zucker, a psychologist and sexologist, is the psychologist-in-chief at Toronto's Centre for Addiction and Mental Health and head of its Gender Identity Service, arguably the world's expert on treating gender dysphoria in children. Dr. Zucker was harassed and silenced by a campaign to discredit his work, led by transgender advocacy groups and transgender-rights activists. Dr. Zucker was slandered because he advocated therapy and a "watch and wait" approach to treating children with gender dysphoria. In his decades of working with children who suffer from gender dysphoria, he discovered that most children's gender dysphoria resolves when they naturally progress through puberty. He noted that trauma and other external factors could cause a child to develop gender dysphoria. Because of this, children with gender dysphoria benefit from therapy in which therapists help a child to understand underlying causes of gender dysphoria.[7]

David Bell, from the Tavistock gender clinic in the UK, was silenced by his superiors and threatened with disciplinary action for voicing concerns about how children with underlying issues were being transed.[8]

Health care professionals who are uncomfortable transing kids are afraid to speak out after witnessing activists' attacks on people like Dr. Zucker, David Bell, and others who have advocated for a watchful waiting approach, rather than embracing the transing model.

However, like most medical and psychiatric conditions, many options exist for treating gender dysphoria.

Therapy can help children resolve or manage their dysphoria so that they are less preoccupied with their feelings of dysphoria. Over time, as underlying emotional struggles are addressed, the dysphoria very often goes away.

All around the world, transgender-rights activists and their gender industry allies are trying to prevent children from accessing therapy as a treatment for gender dysphoria.

Transgender-rights activists and allies forget that the goal should not be to trans children. The goal should be to help these vulnerable children manage or resolve gender dysphoria. But rather than attempt to resolve the gender dysphoria, transgender-rights activists and allies instead prefer to foster it. They want children to focus on their dysphoria, to succumb to it, to accept it as natural.

A doctor does not amputate an arm because a finger has a mild infection. An Al-Anon sponsor doesn't buy booze for an alcoholic instead of encouraging sobriety. We don't give someone with a sprained ankle a wheelchair instead of crutches, and then tell the child she must use the wheelchair for the rest of her life because physical therapy is too much work.

The so-called "affirmative care" model promotes dysfunction over function.

Transing kids is simply abuse.

GENDER?

"So after 4 years of social transition I have realized that I'm not a male, I never was. I transitioned purely because I wanted to not 'have' to deal everything that comes with being a female (shaving, having pretty hair, looking good, dealing with periods, wearing uncomfortable bras...)"

—Posted by PlasticHouseplant*

Sex is a biological reality; each of us is either male or female.

Gender is much more difficult to define, in part because the definition keeps changing. "Gender" originally (and appropriately) applied only to linguistics. Nouns in certain languages were assigned gender (masculine or feminine) which affected their grammatical functions.

Crowdsourced Wikipedia defines gender as "the range of characteristics pertaining to, and differentiating between, masculinity and femininity,"[9] however, historically gender has been used synonymously with sex. Interestingly, trans activists are trying to play both sides of the field with this word. They claim that gender is one's "innermost concept of self as male, female, a blend of both or neither – how individuals perceive themselves and what they call themselves. One's gender identity can be the same or different from their sex assigned at birth,"[10] but then go on to say that one's gender identity determines one's sex.[11]

One can express being a man or a woman in an infinite number of ways. The concept of "gender" really means "personality." No one can legitimately argue that there exists a right or wrong way of being man or a woman. The cultural concept of gender being advanced by activists comprises little more than a bundle of regressive stereotypes.

In fact, people who claim that a female brain can be born into a male body and that a male brain can be born into a female body are simply embracing ridged sex stereotypes.

* * *

Those who are concerned about the trans ideology typically call themselves "gender critical," indicating that they don't believe in the concept of gender as applied to human beings.

In contrast, people who subscribe to gender ideology accept that there is such a thing as a female gender-ness and a male gender-ness that are inherent and innate. They believe that some people are born with their sex and gender-ness matching, but others are born with a mismatch between their sex and gender-ness.

If this is true, then gender roles and stereotypes are created by our gender-ness, in which case, women will always behave as stereotypical females and males will always behave as stereotypical males, unless they are born with a mismatch between their sex and gender-ness.

Not only does this reinforce traditional gender roles and stereotypes, it is also patently untrue.

A woman who does not conform to traditional gender roles is still a woman.

A man who fails to follow stereotypes of masculinity is still male.

Respected evolutionary biologist Heather Heying says, "Gender isn't a human construct, it's not something that we created just for us; it's the behavior that goes along with all of the foundational, anatomical, physiological, chromosomal, genetic you know, stuff that came before."[12]

Regardless of how one views gender, it used to be commonly accepted that *gender* was synonymous with *sex*. Transgender-rights activists have separated gender and sex in confusing and convoluted ways.

They suggest that someone may not actually be the sex they were observed to be at birth; that doctors just "assign" or guess a baby's sex, but the true sex of the child isn't known until the child starts expressing his or her gender.

Huh?

According to this logic, a child's sex is based upon how the child adheres to sex-based stereotypes.

Most rational people find the first problem with this ideology right here.

How someone behaves does not change his or her sex any more than behavior can change age, or place of birth, or eye color.

I can claim to be younger than I am, but that does not make me actually younger. I can put on colored contacts, but that does not change the actual color of my eyes. I can say I was born in Japan, but I was actually born in Salt Lake City. Claiming to be from Japan would simply be a lie.

Those who take the time to analyze transgender ideology quickly recognize that it is flawed, absurd, regressive, and bound up in circular reasoning. Sadly, however most people don't take the time to analyze it. Instead, they swallow the lie that all trans-rights activists want is *tolerance*.

In fact, trans-rights activists want to convince the world that gender and sex are mysteriously intertwined in a mystical way, such that dissonance between the two requires a change in external appearance, often via powerful hormones and surgery.

These medical interventions damage an otherwise healthy body. The actual reality of biology doesn't change, nor does a body's sex change, no matter how many hormones or how much surgery it is subjected to.

* * *

Some argue that cosmetic changes to one's external appearance change one's sex. This is simply not true.

If a penis does not make a man male, then removing it does not make a man female. If breasts do not make a woman female, then having artificial breasts attached to his chest would not make a man female. If the physical characteristics of being female do not make a woman female, then taking hormones to make a male body more look more female does not make a man female.

Our sex is fixed, but the way we express and experience ourselves in our body is constantly changing.

One's experience of one's sexed self is based upon biology, so females will always be women, and males will always be men. A woman who has never had (and never will have) male biology cannot be a man. A man who has never had (and never will have) female biology cannot be a woman.

As University of Manchester researcher Saul McLeod notes, people use to "have very clear ideas about what was appropriate to each sex and anyone behaving differently was regarded as deviant. Today we accept a lot more diversity and see gender as a continuum (*i.e.*, scale) rather than two categories. So men are free to show their 'feminine side' and women are free to show their 'masculine traits.'"[13]

As women gained control over their reproductive lives, traditional gender roles became less important; however the way we interact with the world is still heavily influenced by our biology.

Though sex differences can be somewhat fuzzy around the edges, hundreds of factual differences separate men from women. For example, women are typically smaller and have less muscle mass. Men tend to be larger, with bigger bones and skeletons structurally designed for strength, while women's skeletons are designed for childbirth. Even our hands express sex differences: women's thumbs tend to be longer as compared to the rest of the hand than men's thumbs, and men and women typically have opposite length proportions between their index fingers and ring fingers.

Though the appearance of some of these differences can be manipulated, a woman's body can never become male and a man's body can never become female. When activists make the claim that it is possible to have a male brain in a female body or vice versa, it is nonsensical. In the same way that unusually large feet on a woman does not mean she has male feet, a woman who has characteristics more commonly associated with a male is still a woman.

What determines the sex of our body parts is not feelings or behaviors or actions. What makes a male brain male is being in a male body. What makes a female brain female is being in a female body.

The differences in our experiences are based not on an innate "inner gender" or "gender identity" but on the different ways in which we experience the world as a result of our biological sex differences.

As Heather Heying asserted, our experiences are mediated by our biology.[9]

* * *

Trans-rights activists have coined the term "cis" to refer to anyone who identifies as the sex they were "assigned at birth." This term intends to normalize gender confusion, and those who use it frequently assert that "cis" individuals have no right to any opinions on transgender issues.

Though no definition is ever provided regarding what it means to "identify" as one sex or another, we are all expected to call a "transwoman" a woman, while a biological female is now called a "cis woman."

"Transwomen are women. This is not up for debate—so don't try to," one trans activist reprimanded me.

The entire categories of male and female have been usurped by transgender ideology.

Furthermore, the very notion that doctors simply "assign" the sex of a newborn sends the message to children that their parents and doctor are so ignorant that they can only make a stab-in-the-dark guess about something as fundamental, obvious, and binary as sex categories.

The assertion that doctors merely guess at a baby's sex at birth, is so absurd that one struggles to take the idea seriously. Trans-rights activists further demand that children be raised as "theybies"—without social sex presentation—until the child announces for "theyself" what gender "they be." This would be laughable if it weren't so horrifically damaging to children.

***

When I expressed concern on Facebook about threats of physical violence made by a speaker at a local pro-trans rally, I was told, "So, you don't want to be scared by a speech about standing up to hate, but expect them to be ok living in fear of being attacked or killed? You expect them to just sit back and take it and just preach love and that if they're nice everything will be fine? Is that what you're saying, Erin? Nothing to upset white cis genders like you? Right, Erin?"

This person, who claims to be an LGB & TQ ally, assumed not only that I was "cis," but also that I have no idea what it is like to live in fear. The assumption is that "cis" individuals have never been marginalized or victimized, because "cis" people are too busy oppressing trans people.

Clearly, the term "cis" is not actually used simply to differentiate someone who has not been transed, it is actually used pejoratively against anyone who doesn't identify as transgender. "Cis" is also used to determine who has the right to an opinion and who does not. It determines who has a right to speak and who does not. "Cis" people, therefore, do not have the same freedoms as those who are trans identified, nor should they, according to transgender-rights activists.

Comments like this are ubiquitous: "Let's cut the shit—there's no positive way a cis person can dictate or speak on a life that you do not live and a world you do not have to navigate as a trans person."

Is it any wonder so many children and young adults are adopting a trans identity, when simply being who you were born is now painted as hateful, ignorant, and unworthy of holding an opinion?

"Cis" is a nonsensical term. It is especially problematic when it is applied to those who have struggled with gender dysphoria and either chose not to transition, or who transitioned and then detransitioned.

I do not meet the definition of "cis" gender because I suffer gender dysphoria, but I am not trans because I decided not to remain socially transitioned. Apparently, following the logic of the trans-rights crowd, I don't even exist.

The term "cis" is also problematic for the vast majority of women who experience discomfort in their bodies from time to time, and for the vast majority of kids going through puberty who also feel discomfort in their bodies.

By forcing children to identify their gender based on accepting regressive sexist stereotypes and on the level of comfort they feel with their own bodies, trans-rights activists confuse children into believing that they are not actually the sex they were born.

As concerned parents in Seattle point out, we must take this social engineering seriously, because activists are systematically brainwashing our children to believe that biological sex is an anachronistic term and that we are only what we feel.[14]

Trans-rights activists are inducing gender dysphoria in our children.

* * *

Maria Keffler, my friend and co-host of Commonsense Care, a video series for parents of gender confused kids, often reminds people that gender is nothing more and nothing less than a manifestation of personality.

This becomes obvious as the trans lobby continually expands the ways in which children can identify as transgender, including such absurdities as:

- Abimegender: a gender that is profound, deep, and infinite; meant to resemble when one mirror is reflecting into another mirror creating an infinite paradox
- Cavusgender: for people with depression; when you feel one gender when not depressed and another when depressed
- Espigender: a gender that is related to being a spirit or existing on a higher or extradimensional plane

- Vapogender: a gender that sort of feels like smoke; can be seen on a shallow level but once you go deeper, it disappears and you are left with no gender and only tiny wisps of what you thought it was

Genderspectrum.org claims, "Understandings of gender continually evolve. In the course of a person's life, the interests, activities, clothing, and professions that are considered the domain of one gender or another evolve in ways both small and large."[15]

As it turns out, and as many have observed when trying to make sense of the transgender ideology, there are as many ways to express ourselves as male and female as there are humans on the planet. All of us express ourselves in our own ways, based on our experiences and culture. Now, however, a group of activists insists that the way we express ourselves actually changes our sex.

Those advocating for "affirmative care" (a.k.a. *transing*) are suggesting it is appropriate to change a child's body because the child's personality is one which is stereotypically different from the sex they were born.

Transgender ideology is a profoundly abusive, regressive, and dangerous religion.

GENDER DYSPHORIA

"Every single adult woman can remember a time during her adolescence or maybe her adulthood when the fact that she's female has caused her some distress. And if we are told that that discomfort is an indication that we're actually transgender, we could easily start to kind of inflate those moments and blame our bodies and blame our femalehood for our distress."

—Sasha Ayad
M Ed, LPC[16]

"So as someone who was a victim of the lack of gatekeeping in a sense, I feel I need to speak up personally about this. I literally only ended up transitioning because of my therapist (at the time) suggesting I was a boy in a girl's body because I disliked aspects of being feminine and had an affinity toward masculinity, not to mention my attraction to females. The old gatekeeping systems were based around gender roles."

—Posted by HeavenlyMelody91*

Gender dysphoria can result from a myriad of sources, including trauma, autism, a misunderstanding about gender non-conformity, or subtle messages children pick up from adults or other children. Rather than acknowledging that gender dysphoria is almost always resolved when a child completes puberty naturally, or with the guidance of a good therapist, transgender-rights activists and their allies actively promoting the lie that the only appropriate way to treat a child with gender dysphoria is to encourage them to "transition" to the sex which they identify.

The transing process starts by allowing and encouraging a child to adopt exaggerated stereotypical behaviors and dress of the opposite sex. (Incidentally, this "switch" to espousing the characteristics of the opposite sex only underscores the reality of sex as a binary system.) As a child nears puberty, as young as eight years old, parents are pressured to give their child puberty blockers.

Puberty blockers—the effects of which activists dishonestly claim are reversible—retard a child's normal physical and intellectual maturation.

Following the administration of puberty blockers, the next step in the process is cross-sex hormones. These hormones force a child's body to develop physical characteristics of the opposite sex. Such hormones have significant side effects, infertility being just one.

The final step in transing a child are invasive and extensive surgeries.

Activists have deceived the public to the degree that most people believe that gender confused girls as young as thirteen must have radical mastectomies to remove breast tissue, and both boys and girls as young as sixteen must have surgery to alter their genitals, lest they all commit suicide.

These are lies.

Good therapists don't affirm anorexics who believe they are fat, and they don't advocate gastric bypass surgeries to help anorexics lose more weight. A trustworthy therapist doesn't encourage a hypochondriac who wants his liver removed because he is convinced he has cancer to find a surgeon who will perform the surgery for him. Ethical therapists don't encourage people with obsessive-compulsive disorder to wash their hands until they are raw even if doing so will help them feel like they're clean. Reputable therapists don't agree that patients with paralyzing anxiety are better off never leaving their bedrooms in order to stave off panic attacks. Right-minded therapists don't encourage patients who are cutting themselves to continue to self-harm because it makes them feel good. Adequately trained therapists don't accept and affirm the suicidal ideations of patients who are convinced that life is not worth living.

But today growing numbers of therapists are doing just these things with gender dysphoric patients; in some states they are legally prevented from doing anything else.

The consequences of these "treatments" are staggering.

* * *

Gender dysphoria is a feeling of discomfort or distress that results when someone's feelings about himself or herself conflict with societal expectations and stereotypes regarding how someone of their biological sex should behave.

Gender dysphoria, at its root, is self-hatred. It is also a type of dissociative disorder, which includes "mental disorders that involve experiencing a disconnection and lack of continuity between thoughts, memories, surroundings, actions and identity. People with dissociative disorders escape reality in ways that are involuntary and unhealthy and cause problems with functioning in everyday life."[17]

Ironically, the very definition that is used to justify transing kids—that their feelings of dysphoria are "insistent, persistent, and consistent"—is exactly how healthcare providers assess the seriousness of a mental health issue.[18] Trans-rights activists insist that the more entrenched the dysphoria and dissociation, the more valid the argument that the child was born in the wrong body.

Healthcare providers have long recognized dissociation as a problem to be treated and managed, rather than a lifestyle to be encouraged and embraced.

But that dichotomy has now flipped: doctors and therapists today are pressured to view gender dysphoria as a launch-pad for medicalization, denying the fact that it is in any way a disorder.

What if other disorders were similarly celebrated?

The girl suffering from anorexia nervosa would be offered liposuction and a gastric bypass. The boy with depression would be affirmed that indeed everyone does hate him and his life certainly isn't worth living; he might well be prescribed a lethal dose of morphine. Alcoholic teens might successfully lobby that their high schools install a bar to provide them with easy access to what they feel they desperately need.

Yes, transgender "healthcare" is as ridiculous as it sounds.

* * *

When I suffered from gender dysphoria, my body felt distinctly different from *me*, like I was stuck with something I didn't want. My body caused me a great deal of anger and anxiety. I hated it.

This kind of mental separation from one's body is not healthy.

One's body is part of one's existence, and feelings of alienation from it are red flags that something is terribly wrong, not with our body, but with how we are thinking, feeling, or perceiving ourselves.

Many other mental health issues are characterized by a profound state of unease or dissatisfaction regarding a real or perceived problem. Dysphoria—a state of discomfort or distress—can come in many forms, including:

- major depressive disorder
- bipolar disorder
- borderline personality disorder
- anxiety disorders
- dysphoric rumination
- anxiety disorder
- personality disorders
- body dysmorphic disorder
- schizophrenia
- body integrity dysphoria
- eating disorders

As a society, we recognize that these types of mental health conditions are best treated by managing a person's difficult feelings in order to resolve those feelings. Therapists don't affirm the delusions of a bipolar patient, or the paranoia of a schizophrenic patient, or the anxiety of someone with obsessive-compulsive disorder, because affirming dysphoria exacerbates dysphoria. The more someone focuses their discomfort or distress, the more overwhelming that discomfort or distress becomes.

Gender dysphoria is no different from other types of dysphoria. However, for some reason, it is now supposed to be treated completely differently than any other type of dysphoria: the gender industry insists that it be uncritically, unethically, and irresponsibly affirmed in every single case.

Gender dysphoric children are told that the feelings of distress they have are completely reasonable and appropriate because they are inherently flawed. Somehow they were "born in the wrong body."

Those of us who have experienced gender dysphoria have an appreciation for the many ways that it can develop. Gender identity is based entirely on feelings, and as such, is malleable. Just as our political and religious identities can evolve and change, so too can our gender identity. Likewise, just like our political and religious identities, gender identity is influenced by our experiences and our interpretation of those experiences.

Trauma, comorbid mental illness, autism, ridged understanding of acceptable gender roles and behavior can all manifest as gender dysphoria. But the idea that "gender" is somehow biological, fixed, or innate is unsupported by science and wholly absurd.

* * *

The idea that gender dysphoria should be affirmed is relatively new. Transgender-rights activists have mounted a successful campaign to normalize and then medicalize gender dysphoria. Using misinformation, pseudo-science, and false information, transgender-rights activists have convinced many that gender dysphoria is biological, and that an actual mismatch can exist between someone's internal sense of gender and their outward biological sex.

George Orwell coined the term "newspeak" and "doublespeak" to refer to the way language can be manipulated for political purposes. Orwell's landmark novel *1984* chronicles the dangers of totalitarianism, and how totalitarians use language to obscure reality as a way of controlling society.[19] Trans-rights activists have become masters at obfuscating language in exactly the way Orwell predicted in his book.

Trans-rights activists have changed how we talk about something as basic as the recording of a child's sex at birth. Trans-rights activists insist that babies are "assigned" a sex at birth. No, they're not. Babies are not "assigned" a sex at birth; children are born male or female. Just as the birthdate and time of birth are factual bits of data, so is the sex of the newborn.

These facts of birth are recorded, not assigned.

Mainstream providers of health information are largely unwilling to acknowledge that gender dysphoria is a mental health issue, because transgender-rights activists have been so effective at promoting misinformation and disinformation about gender dysphoria. In doing so, these activists and providers further stigmatize mental illness by performing all kinds of contortions of reason in order to prove that gender dysphoria is not a mental health issue.

However, in order to get treatment and file insurance claims for medical interventions, some kind of diagnosis is required.

The American Psychiatric Association currently claims that gender dysphoria in and of itself is not a mental health problem. Rather, the distress caused by an unsupportive and intolerant society is assigned blame for any feelings of distress experienced by someone who suffers gender dysphoria.[20] In order to address this "unsupportive" and "intolerant" society, those with gender dysphoria have to change their external appearance often with extreme interventions, in order to alleviate the distress they have.

This explanation is so convoluted and illogical it is difficult to follow, let alone believe.

* * *

The idea that gender stems from biology makes no sense. Gender stereotypes (like "boys play football" and "girls are scared of bugs") are socially constructed. Gender norms change throughout history as well as across cultures because they are based on societal expectations.

To suggest that gender, and more specifically gender dysphoria is biologically determined would be like claiming that someone with anorexia nervosa was biologically programed to feel fat in a skinny body, or that someone with obsessive-compulsive disorder was born in a body that is chromosomally germophobic.

This line of reasoning blames the body for the mental health disorder, rather than accepting the logical and sensible conclusion that dysphoria – or a feeling of discomfort with oneself – originates in the way the mind interprets the body's experiences.

Those advocating such an irrational and untenable position often bully and harass anyone who disagrees with their strange perspective. Why? Because it is far easier to intimidate others into acceptance of affirmative care than to prove the benefits of "affirmative care," since it's unclear that "affirmative care" actually provides any benefits.

* * *

Dr. Kenneth Zucker, one of the first clinicians to pioneer treatment for children with gender dysphoria, advocated either a watchful-waiting approach or talk therapy. He noted that trauma and other external factors can cause a child to develop gender dysphoria. Therefore, he noted, children with gender dysphoria benefit greatly from therapy that helps them manage or resolve their dysphoria.[21, 22] Over decades of working with children who suffered from gender dysphoria, Dr. Zucker discovered that most children's gender dysphoria resolves simply by progressing naturally through puberty.

But transgender advocacy groups and activists targeted Dr. Zucker with harassment, censorship, and by discrediting his work because he did not fall in line with their demands for an affirmation-only response to gender dysphoria. Transgender-rights activists don't want to accept Dr. Zucker's professional, experienced, and research-supported treatment plan, even though children who are encouraged to socially transition and then to medically transition have exorbitantly high rates of mental illness.

The transgender community blames poor psychiatric outcomes on social harassment and discrimination, rather than accepting the well-documented fact that transitioning sexes does not solve mental health issues.[23]

To bolster their claims that society's harassment, discrimination and violence against transgender-identified people are responsible for the outrageously poor mental health outcomes of those who transition, transgender-rights activists have expanded the definition of "violence": included today are *misgendering* (using the "wrong" pronouns to address a transgender individual) and *deadnaming* (using a person's birth name).[24] According to trans-rights activists, saying a single word someone else doesn't prefer is tantamount to murder.

Trans-rights activists utilize other tricks of language and alternate definitions to convince people that transgender individuals are the victims of harassment, violence, and discrimination. They must resort to such subterfuge in order to justify the spurious claim that the reason transitioned individuals continue to have mental health issues is not because of underlying mental health issues, but because of how society treats those who have transed.[25]

* * *

Affirming gender dysphoria, teaching children that they are victims of abuse if someone uses the wrong pronoun, and encouraging kids to feel like they are oppressed are not ways to promote emotional wellbeing.

Transing promotes disease over health, because once someone medically transitions, s/he will almost certainly have lifelong side effects and complications.[26] People who have attempted to transition sexes nearly always experience worsened physical and psychological health.[27]

A survey for those who transitioned and then detransitioned found that a myriad of conditions and experiences lead to gender dysphoria.[28] This survey also found, as one would expect, that transitioning did not resolve the underlying causes of the gender dysphoria. Rather, transitioning encourages a gender dysphoric person to run away from him- or herself, and to create a new persona, without ever addressing the desire to escape oneself in the first place.

We don't actually need a survey to tell us that underlying mental health issues cause gender dysphoria; simply listening to detransitioners provides critical insights.

I'm a detransitioner. In my case and in so many others, the cause of my gender dysphoria was a sexual assault.

Sexual Assault

During the summer before I entered first grade, my brother and I were abducted by two men and taken to a public restroom. I was brutally sexually assaulted, while my brother was not.

In my child's mind, I thought that being a boy would prevent me from ever being hurt again in the way those men hurt me.

No one initially knew that I'd made that erroneous determination. Neither my mother, nor my school teacher, nor my school psychologist recognized that the sudden appearance of my "trans" identity resulted from my desire to prevent being sexually violated again. It took years of therapy before I came to understand the connection.

If therapists had affirmed my gender dysphoria, I never would have come to understand that my hatred of my female body was the direct result of my female body being violently violated. Had I been "affirmed," I never would have realized that my trans identity was a coping mechanism.

I am so thankful that my school psychologist put me on a healing path.

I am grateful to other therapists who helped me understand that my self-hatred resulted from the sexual assault, not because I was inherently flawed.

I shudder to think what my life would be like had I been encouraged to believe that I was born in the wrong body. I would have lived my life hating myself. I would have taken puberty blockers and then cross-sex hormones that would likely have rendered me sterile, and caused my body to become dysfunctional. I would have had my healthy breasts amputated as soon as I could find a surgeon to do it.

If I were the only child who developed gender dysphoria as a result of a sexual assault, it would be enough to dispel trans-rights activists' insistence that a child "knows" his or her gender identity, that gender identity is fixed, and that children with gender dysphoria are born in the wrong body.

But I am not the only one.

In his article, *Childhood Sexual Abuse, Gender Dysphoria, and Transition Regret: Billy's Story*, detransitioner Walt Heyer writes, "The shame and pain of being used by a sexual predator is beyond the imagination. Most abused kids push the feelings deep inside and shut out the memories. The pain, shame, guilt, and fear often keep them from telling anyone about the abuse until much later in life, if they ever do. Many sexual abuse victims—like Billy, me, and others who write to me—get swept up by LGBT therapists who suggest that the proper treatment is to start on powerful sex hormones followed by gender 'affirming' surgery. The problem is that hormones and surgery will not be effective in providing long-term treatment for depression or other ailments caused by sexual trauma."[29]

Children who are sexually abused often blame their bodies—and specifically their genitals—for what happened to them. Often, as in my case, this is all done subconsciously. It takes a good trauma therapist to help extricate those beliefs.

The *Transgender Victims of Sexual Assault* report states "The vast majority of transgender sexual assault survivors who responded to FORGE's 2005 survey were first assaulted as children or youth."[30]

One survivor wrote, "I had no sense of self but I knew I didn't want to be a woman because bad things happen to women. I developed a very masculine self at a young age after being raped, and it was absolutely to dissociate myself from pain."

Another responded, "I...feel that my experiences of sexual abuse massively impacted my ability to tolerate my presence within my body, and my relationship to the material consequences of operating this body."

Someone else stated, "PTSD - raped by a girl at 19...Needed anything to show me a way out of my body. Anything to make it not the body that could be hurt by someone else."[31]

YouTuber Elle Palmer said, "I had just gone through a very traumatic sexual experience with an older man," right before she developed gender dysphoria.[32]

It is unconscionable that healthcare providers are overlooking the trauma and feelings of dissociation from the body that survivors—especially childhood survivors—of sexual assault experience.

Trans-rights activists know about this connection. They know that many kids who claim a trans identity have had their small bodies violated in unthinkable ways. They know that transing these kids is encouraging them to temporarily run away from the pain of trauma, and that transing these kids does not heal them.

Transing tells kids that the shame they feel is justified.

Transing gives people the message that they shouldn't talk about what happened.

Transing encourages children to run away from themselves.

Transing celebrates burying trauma deep inside.

Autism

Children with autism are increasingly encouraged to believe they are transgender.

In her article *12 Causes of Gender Dysphoria*, Melinda Selmys observed, "Women with Asperger's and other autism spectrum conditions often report that they find it easier to interact with males, and to fit in in male society. Some of the common symptoms of autism (lack of social awareness, a tendency towards more logical forms or abstracted forms of thought) may be experienced as 'masculine.' Autistic people are also often asexual and may have a complicated relationship with their bodies. On a purely anecdotal level, I've found that gender-atypical presentations seem to be more common with autistic friends than among neurotypical folks."[33]

One of the clinicians at a gender clinic reported the concern, "Maybe we're medicating kids with autism."[34] Rather than performing a full diagnostic assessment of children who came to the clinic, it was assumed the children were transgender.

Why?

Because current diagnostic criteria demands that a kid be transed if the kid simply says he or she is trans.[35]

Thankfully, not every clinic takes this approach. Nem went to a gender clinic in Scotland. Rather than automatically transing her, they gave her a full assessment and diagnosed her with autism. Once she started getting help to manage her autism, she realized that her gender dysphoria was related to both her autism as well as a prior sexual assault.[36] Had she gone to an affirmation-only clinic, she likely would have been transed rather than getting the help she needed to sort out how the combination of trauma and autism led to her gender dysphoria.

It makes sense that children—especially girls with autism—might come to believe that they are male, because autism interferes with social skills. Girls are expected to have good social skills, and girls who lack social skills are often ostracized.

One autistic female subject from the *Female Detransition and Reidentification* study mentioned earlier said, "My autism made me see other females as a completely different species." [32]

Ashira, who was diagnosed with autism after she detransitioned, said, "I think that as a kid, it was difficult for me to communicate in general in terms of like my feelings and my inner world could not communicate. So having some way to identify what was wrong was a reason that I, what do you call it, turned to transgenderism."[37]

According to the Center for Disease Control, about one in fifty-four children has been identified with autism spectrum disorder.[38] Yet the rates of kids being transed who are on the autism spectrum is outrageously higher. The study, *Clinical Presentations and Challenges Experienced by a Multidisciplinary Team and Gender Service* found that nearly 14% of the children being transed were diagnosed with autism.[39] Considering that boys are four times more likely to be diagnosed with autism than girls, but more girls were represented in their study, this is an alarming rate.

Another study reports that 24% of those who have transed have been diagnosed with autism.[40]

Once again, trans-rights activists are encouraging children with developmental issues to trans, rather than providing them support to help them function.

It will be incredibly difficult for kids with autism to process what was done to them by healthcare professionals who gave them the false impression that they would be cured by transing.

Attention Deficit Hyperactivity Disorder (ADHD)

Children, and especially girls, who are diagnosed with attention deficit/hyperactivity disorder (ADHD) are also susceptible to gender dysphoria. Hyper boys are more culturally acceptable, while girls are expected to be quiet and compliant.

Two participants in the detransition study commented on their experience with ADHD:

"I'd always felt like I had a male brain and I think it had heavily to do with my inability to relate to other females due to pretty severe ADHD."

"My alienation from femaleness was related in part to how ADD [attention deficit disorder] features made me unable to meet the gendered expectations (behaviorally and aesthetically) others had for me."

In his study on the links between ADHD and gender identity, John Strang of the Children's National Medical Center in Washington, DC found, "Children and teenagers with an autism spectrum disorder or those who have attention deficit and hyperactivity problems are much more likely to wish to be another gender."[41]

Transing these kids provides a temporary solution to what might not even be gender dysphoria, but rather a desperate attempt to fit in with their peers.

Depression and Anxiety

Depression and anxiety can create feelings of gender dysphoria. Detransitioners often address the connection between depression, anxiety, and gender dysphoria:

"My dysphoria certainly fed my depression and vice versa, pushing me to identify as a trans man and look into transitioning."

"I felt that because I was depressed and wanted to escape my body that transition would help solve all my problems."

"I feel like anxiety worsened by vitriolic 2013 Tumblr discourse kinda... made me, an impressionable kid, feel like I was a bad person if I wasn't trans."[42]

Medications that are used for depression and anxiety often short circuit a teen's sexual development. As other young people are having their first twinges of sexual desire, teens on antidepressants and antianxiety medications either may not develop a sex drive, or may find that their previously developing sex drive has shut down.

Parents might feel an understandable sense of relief that they needn't worry about their teenagers becoming sexually active, but sexual development is an integral part of human development. Derailing sexual maturation does no service to the young person. Kids who don't experience sexual interest might feel like they are even more different from their peers, exacerbating the problems further.

Here we find one more possible disconnect from the body, and yet another opportunity to trans vulnerable kids.

Eating Disorders

Children with eating disorders and other types of body dysmorphia can also experience feelings of gender dysphoria.[43] This shouldn't be a surprise, since eating disorders result from blaming one's body for one's problems. This excessive focus on the body results in a generalized dysphoria and a disconnect between the body and the mind. People suffering body dysmorphic disorders feel like they are in the wrong body, as described by these two detransitioners:

"...Body Dysmorphic Disorder was often misconstrued with Dysphoria, as I constantly felt my body was 'wrong,' and felt less so when not performing femininity."

"I confused my body dysmorphia, brought on by the pressure to be thin, small and beautiful and worsened by my anorexia, with dysphoria. I thought that the only way I could be happy being large and strong and obnoxious and taking up space was by being male."[43]

I have been amazed at the number of detransitioners who struggle with eating disorders, but the issue does sound familiar. As my own body started to mature, I experienced extreme discomfort with the changes that betrayed my desire to be perceived as male. I began to diet and purge to try to force my body to retain its pre-pubescent androgyny.

When I watch interviews of Ellen Page (who announced to the world on December 1, 2020 that she was actually a man) I wonder if she also suffered an eating disorder. She appears skeletal, and despondent. Shortly after Page's big announcement, she had her breasts removed. As she shared her feelings of distress prior to her mastectomy, it leads one to wonder if she viewed her breasts as the last remaining fat on her body that needed to be excised.

Doctors who would never agree to remove fat from an anorexic patient willingly chop breasts off of anorexic girls and women who think they are transgender.

Once again those with significant mental health issues are being told that transing is the solution, reinforcing the self-hatred they have and enabling them to run away from themselves rather than resolve their underlying issues.

Rapid Onset Gender Dysphoria

In her article, *Outbreak: On Transgender Teens and Psychic Epidemics*, Lisa Marchiano discusses "psychic outbreaks" and "social contagions."

Currently, we appear to be experiencing a significant psychic epidemic that is manifesting as children and young people coming to believe that they are the opposite sex, and in some cases taking drastic measures to change their bodies. Of particular concern to the author is the number of teens and tweens suddenly coming out as transgender without a prior history of discomfort with their sex. "Rapid-onset gender dysphoria" is a new presentation of a condition that has not been well studied. Reports online indicate that a young person's coming out as transgender is often preceded by increased social media use and/or having one or more peers also come out as transgender. These factors suggest that social contagion may be contributing to the significant rise in the number of young people seeking treatment for gender dysphoria.[44]

A Brown University study found that 'rapid-onset gender dysphoria' (ROGD) may be a social contagion linked with an increase in internet use, an identity politics culture, and having friends who identify as LGBT. In her study, *Rapid-onset gender dysphoria in adolescents and young adults: A study of parental reports*, Lisa Littman found that "Rapid-onset gender dysphoria (ROGD) describes a phenomenon where the development of gender dysphoria is observed to begin suddenly during or after puberty in an adolescent or young adult who would not have met criteria for gender dysphoria in childhood. ROGD appears to represent an entity that is distinct from the gender dysphoria observed in individuals who have previously been described as transgender."[45]

Littman also found that ROGD was common in children who ascribed to a neo-Marxist view of privilege. "In general, cis-gendered people are considered evil and unsupportive, regardless of their actual views on the topic. To be heterosexual, comfortable with the gender you were assigned at birth, and non-minority, places you in the 'most evil' of categories with this group of friends. Statement of opinions by the evil cis-gendered population are consider phobic and discriminatory and are generally discounted as unenlightened."

One of the detrans survey respondents said, "I believe that social anxiety and the desire to 'fit in' with the QSA (Queer-Straight Alliance) at my school--almost all non-binary or FTM women--led to my decision to identify as nonbinary."[46]

It isn't surprising that white, middle class children who would otherwise be considered the most privileged (or in their minds, most evil) would have a desire to opt out of their identity. Transing allows them to change from being considered the oppressor to being marginalized and oppressed.

It is unimaginable that we are transing children with dangerous and experimental interventions rather than helping them learn to manage their difficult feelings. These kids are being damaged physically. They are being given the message that they are not capable of dealing with difficult feelings and that running away from oneself is the only solution. This strategy of escape can only result in dysfunction until children realize that they are capable of sorting through problems and working through uncomfortable feelings.

Abigail Shrier's fantastic exposé explains how girls with rapid onset gender dysphoria are being encouraged to transition, rather than being taught to manage the difficult feelings associated with adolescence. As Shrier says, "The psychological struggles that lead a young woman to transition are often acute." She also notes that "the new 'affirmative-care' standard of mental health professionals is a different matter entirely. It surpasses sympathy and leaps straight to demanding that mental health professionals adopt their patients' beliefs of being in the 'wrong body.' Affirmative therapy compels therapists to endorse a falsehood: not that a teenage girl feels more comfortable presenting as a boy—but that she actually is a boy."[47]

* * *

With all these obvious and well-researched underlying causes of gender dysphoria, why would an affirmative care model, which encourages gender dysphoria, be adopted? Why are so few healthcare professionals asking this very question? Why do trans-rights advocates attack with slurs and silencing campaigns when someone dares to question the affirmation-only narrative?

Jennifer Bilek has gone deep and wide to explore the motivations behind transing kids. Her website, *The 11th Hour Blog*, offers frightening insights into how children's vulnerabilities are being leveraged by big pharma and other business interests in order to make millions of dollars via transing young people. Bilek has followed the money and uncovered the hideous underbelly of the gender industry.[48] "Over the past decade, there has been an explosion in transgender medical infrastructure across the United States and world to 'treat' transgender people. In addition to gender clinics proliferating across the United States, hospital wings are being built for specialized surgeries, and many medical institutions are clamoring to get on board with the new developments."

It is hard to imagine that anyone would push healthy children toward medications and surgery that damage them for life, when these children could be taught how to manage their difficult feelings without any need for medications or surgery.

And yet, all the evidence tells us that this is exactly what is happening.

TRANSING AWAY THE GAY

"I'm a profoundly unhappy male with unresolved childhood traumas who transitioned as a way to escape myself and I did believe I'm trans but I'm probably just a very effeminate looking/acting guy. Have little to do with the community because I'm attacked for not being supportive of transition, for having doubts, for having thought crimes."

—Posted by ICQME*

How did the "T" get added to "LGB," anyway?

Sexual orientation relates to whom someone finds sexually attractive.

Transgenderism refers to a perceived disconnect between body and mind, which is better understood as gender dysphoria.

Sexual orientation and gender dysphoria have exactly nothing in common.

Personality—what trans-rights activists call "gender expression"—is not a sexual orientation, and should not be treated as one. Even the concept of gender expression is problematic, suggesting that our sex is inextricably connected to our clothing, how we wear our hair, or the kinds of things we like to do. In other words, we are held hostage by our sex, or (in the gender industry's vernacular) our "gender expression."

Because transgender ideology insists that our sex changes according to one's gender expression, it is impossible to know if some kind of gender spirit overrides our sex, or if our sex is undermined by this supposed gender spirit. Either way, this ephemeral "spirit," which is impossible to quantify, define, isolate, or explain, exerts enormous power over us, according to trans-rights activists.

A growing number of LGB groups and individuals are attempting to extricate themselves from the TQAI++ (of LGBTQAI++), wondering how it took hold of their community in the first place. YouTuber and gay man Menno expressed concern that he very likely would have been transed if he were a kid today.[49]

Andrea O'Brien, a lesbian, also believes that she would have been transed were she a child today. "When I was eleven, I used to pray to God every day to be made Andrew, so that I could date girls. I would have 100% been transed had I been born ten years later."[50]

Additionally, concerns are increasing that transing is actually an insidious form of conversion therapy that is being adopted by communities that otherwise would consider themselves tolerant and supportive of those who are lesbian, gay, and bisexual. Children who might grow up to be gay or lesbian are being told they are born in the wrong body. Even the American Psychiatric Associations Diagnostic and Statistical Manual notes that many children who suffer from gender dysphoria grow up to be gay or lesbian.[51]

But if children are transed, they will never have that opportunity. If they transition sexes, it seems, they magically transition from gay to straight.

* * *

In Iran, gay men are given the option to transition (to appear to look like a woman) or go to prison and sometimes even be put to death.[52] Though the pressure in other places may not be this overt, countless cases emerge where parents of effeminate boys decide their son is actually a girl who was born in the wrong body. Is this simply a preemptive homophobic response to a son who is not behaving as they think he should? Parents of a tomboy who worry their little girl is showing signs of being a lesbian, may tell her she is actually a boy; teachers, doctors, and mental health care providers subsequently assure her that her parents are right.

A teen girl who is just starting to experience arousal by same sex peers might decide she is actually a boy in order to avoid the label of lesbian.

A young man who has been teased for being a "sissy" his whole life might decide that it will be easier living as a girl.

I have spoken to older lesbians and gays who freely admit that if they were children today they might trans to avoid the stigma of being homosexual. Detransitioner Sydney Wright has become an important voice for lesbians. She says it was internalized homophobia that caused her to trans. "In my mind, the people that were the transgenders, they were walking the streets with their girlfriend or loved one. Nobody knew that they were actually gay."[53]

But transing did not turn out well for her.

Sydney told Alabama legislators, "Two years ago, I was a healthy, beautiful teenage girl heading toward high school graduation. But after taking testosterone for a year, I turned into an overweight, pre-diabetic nightmare of a transgender 'man.'"[54]

* * *

Scott Newgent was a lesbian before transing.

Scott explains:

> I fell in love with somebody that was a very, very devout Catholic, very, very devout Catholic. And unfortunately her family did not accept homosexuality at all. And, so when we got together, I was kind of known as the lesbian devil, but nobody ever met me. They never saw pictures of me. So I kind of was going through that process when Jenner was transitioning. And I just said, you know what I've always thought about? It seems like it would fix the solution. It seems like a Disney fairytale. Well, why don't we give it a shot?[55]

For Scott and others, the reality of transitioning proved not a fairytale, but a nightmare. Scott experienced life-threatening medical complications and was left physically damaged and emotionally ravaged.

Scott isn't the only one speaking out as children are being encouraged to transition.

Effeminate boys and masculine girls may develop gender dysphoria because of their parents' homophobia. Believing that gender is defined by external stereotypically gendered behaviors and preferences, the parents may prefer a straight child of the opposite sex to a gay child of the sex that was born to them.

Kai Shappley's mother, Kimberly Shappley, admits in a documentary that she was terrified her son was gay. She said "we started praying fervently," and that she even Googled conversion therapy. When she learned about "trans kids," suddenly her gay boy was no longer gay, but a girl born in the wrong body.[56]

Some trans-affirming parents say they "knew" from the time their child was young, even before eight years old—and sometimes before the child was even born—that the child was transgender.

In the BBC documentary *Transgender Kids: Who Knows Best*, one parent admits to being more accepting of his effeminate son after he transitioned. The father said that after transitioning, he was so happy watching his "daughter" run, because as a father, he could say "that is my daughter running like a girl," instead of cringing as he watched his "son run like a girl."

As another parent in the same documentary said, "It is easier for her to just be a girl, than to be a gay boy."[57]

In fact, videos of parents talking about their gender non-conforming child are ubiquitous on YouTube these days. Most of these parents say something like, "I knew from the time my daughter was five that she was meant to be a man," or "it has always been clear that my son was supposed to be a girl."

Often these parents say they "knew" because their child liked toys typically associated with the opposite gender or they liked to dress up in clothes of the opposite gender. Perhaps their child had mannerisms associated with the opposite gender.

Amber Briggle, an outspoken advocate of medically transitioning children, stated in a *TED Talk* that she knew her daughter was actually a boy because her daughter told her while still in-utero that she was really a boy.[58]

Concerns brought forward by whistleblowers about the Tavistock clinic in the U.K. specifically state that clinicians were concerned they were transing gay kids.

In a special report for *BBC Newsnight*, investigative journalist Debrah Cohen said, "Some parents appeared to prefer the child was transgender and straight rather than gay, pushing them towards transition."

One clinician said, "Maybe we are medicating gay kids."

Another concerned staff member said, "We did have a lot of families and parents who would actively tell us that, 'Oh, I'm so glad, at least my child is not gay or lesbian,' implying that having a trans outcome would be better for their children."[59]

It seems that if parents are uncomfortable with a feminine boy or a masculine girl, they can easily nudge their child toward gender confusion today, especially if those children are sensitive and want to please their parents.

When parents like Rep. Marie Newman say that the day her child adopted a trans identity was the happiest day of her life, it seems clear the child wasn't fully acceptable to the parents prior to transing.[60]

* * *

Another staff member from the Tavistock gender clinic admitted, "I had a case. There was a lot of trauma in the family. The young person had come out initially as a lesbian and had faced a lot of homophobic bullying, both very subtly within the family and quite openly in school. And suddenly the young person changed their mind and they started identifying as trans."[61]

Lisa Wilson, a lesbian social worker, said "I find it disheartening that all of our tomboy, butch and 'masculine' females are being told that they must be a male simply because they don't fit the stereotype of what a female 'should' be. This ideology is being promoted in the name of progress but it is truly regressive for women's rights."[62]

Is the push to put children on puberty blockers and transition them with surgery and hormones before they are even adults really about *acceptance,* or is it actually nothing but an insidious form of homophobia?

Though these children might grow up to be gay, this concern is based in regressive beliefs about stereotypical behavior and the lack of acceptance for gender non-conforming children. It also may indicate deep-seated homophobia that is projected on gender non-conforming children.

In other words, transing kids is just another form of conversion therapy.

AUTOGYNEPHILIA

"But there are guys like me and the word 'autogynephilia' although I can't say I've been diagnosed with that or anything, I read up on it and there are men who get more of a sexual kick of being, not looking like a woman, but living as a woman. And that word autogynephilia, that gets shunned and demonized by so many transgender-rights activists. But I honestly believe that's there needs to be more research into it. Me, I like women and so if anything, for me, it's like, I think beautiful women are hot. So the hottest thing would be if I was a beautiful woman."

—Josh Drews[63]

"It just got to the point where enough is enough. I'm just a dude in a dress."

—Kevin[64]

An autogynephile is a male who becomes sexually aroused by the thought of himself as a female. Autogynephilia is sometimes conflated with gender dysphoria, but these two disorders are not at all the same thing.

First identified by Sexologist Ray Blanchard his book *The Man Who Would Be Queen*, autogynephilia is a paraphilia, or disorder of one's sexuality. Blanchard noted that the autogynephile (AGP) typically doesn't have surgery to invert his penis because he enjoys being sexually aroused as a man.[65]

Autogynephilic men often do, however, want breast augmentation surgery. In the words of one AGP, "I am a boob guy and like, so whenever I get the urge to touch a boob, I can just touch my own."[66]

* * *

In her article, *Autogynephilia: An Underappreciated Paraphilia*, Professor of Psychology A.A. Lawrence found that "Nearly 3% of men in Western countries may experience autogynephilia."[5]

Three percent is an astonishingly high rate of occurrence. This number could explain why such a push exists to normalize a sexual fetish that objectifies women's bodies for sexual gratification.

AGPs adopt what many consider to be harmful and stereotypical ideals of woman. These sexually disordered men attempt to appropriate womanhood for themselves by insisting that they magically become women just because they "feel" like women.

Rather, they are using this narrative to gain access to women-only spaces in order to indulge their sexual fetish.

* * *

Miranda Yardley, a transexual male, discusses four different variations of autogynephilia:

- Transvestic autogynephilia: arousal to the act or fantasy of wearing typically feminine clothing
- Behavioral autogynephilia: arousal to the act or fantasy of doing something regarded as feminine
- Physiologic autogynephilia: arousal to fantasies of body functions specific to people regarded as female
- Anatomic autogynephilia: arousal to the fantasy of having a normative woman's body, or parts of one[67]

The AGP does not feel he is born in the wrong body; rather he has a paraphilia and gets sexually aroused at the idea of himself being female.

* * *

Anyone who spends much time around AGPs realizes that these men mimic how they perceive women's behavior; but as they try hard to impersonate women, their maleness shows through. They may insist that the only reason they want to use a woman's restroom is to "pee," but those of us who have had the unpleasant experience of sharing a bathroom with an AGP know this is not true.

The AGP struts into the bathroom as if he owns the place, daring someone to challenge his right to be there. He does not avert his eyes as the women in the bathroom change or adjust their clothes. He is not there to pee; he is there to colonize a woman's space because it turns him on to do so.

As blogger Nina Paley said, this is about the "literal occupation of women's spaces – rape shelters, prisons, locker rooms, bathrooms, swimming holes, and women-only events that women have fought very hard for. By men. Physically."[68]

One of the very common responses an AGP gives when told he is not actually a woman is "suck my dick" or "choke on my dick" or some other variation of verbalization of sexual violence against the woman he is addressing.[69]

Though these men objectify women for their own sexual pleasure, there needs to be compassion for boys and teens struggling with autogynephilia. Rather than getting help to manage their fetish, they too are being transed. Often these boys have been groomed into autogynephilia by sissy-hypno porn.

One man describes this type of porn: "Hypnosis media that turn participants into sexy, cocksucking sissies."[70]

It is hard to find information about sissy-hypno porn because when Googling it, the first of hundreds of hits link to actual porn.

Graham Lineham, writer of popular TV shows *The IT Crowd*, *Black's Books*, and *Father Ted* wrote an article about sissy-hypno porn because he felt it important to report on "the phenomenon of pornography-induced dysphoria that simultaneously promotes extreme sexual objectification and the degradation of womanhood."

Sissy-hypno porn, Lineham says, "typically involves men wearing lingerie and engaged in 'forced feminization' – eroticizing the illusion of being made to 'become women' through dress, makeup, and sexual submissiveness, and the fetishizing of the humiliation this brings."[71]

Andrea Long Chu says in his book *Females* that "Sissy porn's central conceit is that the women it depicts are in fact former men who have been feminized ('sissified') by being forced to wear makeup, wear lingerie, and perform acts of sexual submission. Captions further instruct viewers to understand that the very act of looking at sissy porn itself constitutes an act of sexual degradation, with the implication that, whether they like it or not, viewers will inevitably be transformed into females themselves."[72]

These are boys and young men who have had their sexuality highjacked. Though it may be difficult to see them as victims because their behavior can be so abhorrent, they are in need of support to help them reclaim both their sexuality as well as their identity as male.

SUICIDE

Transgender-rights activists parrot *ad nauseum* the propaganda that if kids are not transed, they will kill themselves:

- If everyone doesn't use a transed child's new name, he will kill himself.
- If everyone doesn't use a transed child's preferred pronouns, she will kill herself.
- If transed children are not allowed to wear the clothes they want, they will kill themselves.
- If transed children are not allowed to get the haircuts they want, they will kill themselves.
- If transed children are not allowed to use the opposite sex's bathroom, they will kill themselves.
- If transed children are not allowed to compete in the opposite sex's sports, they will kill themselves.

And of course, if transed kids are not allowed access to all the medical interventions they want, they will kill themselves. These medical interventions include puberty blockers, cross sex hormones, and surgeries.

Parents of daughters are told, "You can have a dead daughter or a live son."

Parents of sons are told, "You can have a live daughter or a dead son."

Threats of suicide are not only emotional blackmail, they are also potentially incredibly dangerous. Such propaganda communicates to children that if they don't get what they want, the appropriate response is suicide. It trains them to manipulate others to get what they want, and it also puts children in danger of self-harm.

Just as transing is a social contagion, so is suicide. In other words, telling children they will kill themselves is likely to result in children killing themselves.[73]

Children should never be taught, told, encouraged, or in any way led to believe that suicide is an appropriate response to any of life's challenges. To do so would be to embrace suicide as an option. If it is an option, the likelihood of children attempting and completing suicide will increase. Instead, children need to be taught that they can handle difficult feelings.

Activists propagate wild lies about transing interventions being "lifesaving medical treatment," when, in fact, the data shows exactly the opposite.

As Dr. Kevin Stuart, executive director of the Austin Institute for the Study of Family & Culture reports, "multiple studies have shown that over the long run, those who transition have increased rates of suicidality, not decreased."[74]

* * *

Susie Green, the CEO of Mermaids (an organization that pushes children's transition) and a mother who transed her own teenage son, makes the outrageous statement that transing kids "is literally lifesaving treatment" and that any efforts to regulate it will result in "the inevitable rise in self-harm and suicide."[75]

This abusive and untrue narrative launched decades ago via doctors like Stanley Beber[76] and Norman Spack,[77] who first pushed the absurd notion that something akin to a gender spirit could accidentally be housed in the wrong body. This belief has gained traction over the years as more and more adherents have joined the transgender movement.

The claims from those pushing this narrative are prolific, unsubstantiated, and bizarre.

The ACLU claims, "Gender-affirming care is medically necessary care that can be life-saving for transgender youth."[78]

Dr. Elizabeth Miller claims, "My sense is cross-sex hormones, pubertal blockers are absolutely medically necessary."[79]

Dr. Colton Wasserman says, "It's vital for trans people, especially young trans people, to access the supportive, affirming health care *they* choose."[80]

Dr. Michelle Forcier makes the absurd assertion that, "Puberty blockers are safe and effective and this is totally reversible," and as such, "it is sort of a no-brainer to make these available."[81]

Activist Max Mowitz says, "Gender-affirming care is lifesaving and essential."[82]

Dr. Keith Hansen testified that medically transing children, "has demonstrated significant reductions in suicidal ideation, suicide, depression, anxiety, and self-harm."[83]

In fact, however, the very opposite is true.[84, 85, 86]

Bev Jackson from the LGB Alliance is alarmed about what amounts to calculated lies by those pushing the medicalization of gender dysphoric kids, saying it is "very unfortunate, false suicide statistics that are bantered about." She goes on to say, "I think this is so irresponsible, and what you want when you have children in distress is to find out what the causes are of their distress."[87]

It is horrific that so many medical professionals would rather push children onto a regime of experimental drugs, which come with significant risks and side effects, than to explore the real, underlying issues causing the child's distress.

* * *

Though we don't yet have any valid longitudinal data on children who have been transed, all of the credible and professional research suggests that over the long term, those who transition have poor outcomes.[88]

Dr. Patrick Lappert laments, "Parents are being bullied into believing that the risk of suicide is so great that they must accept all these terrible effects. This is not true. The only solid long-term data in a population study that is not biased by the sampling errors and short follow up, shows us that persons who have completed all of the medical and surgical treatments have a suicide rate that is nineteen times higher than matched controls."[89]

Such numbers are staggering. Based on the longitudinal study Lappert cites, transing actually increases the likelihood that a child will die by suicide.

Not only do activists harm children by encouraging the suicide narrative, there have even been instances of mental health professionals encouraging children to fake a suicide attempt in order to medically transition.

Canadian psychologist Dr. Wallace Wong, who makes a comfortable living by encouraging kids to transition, was captured on tape saying, "Pull a stunt. Suicide every time. They will give you what you need."[90]

Dr. Andre Van Mol explains, "Therapists and doctors are being brow-beaten. In fact, bullied, you know that, 'Hey, you either support transition or it's suicide.' And the classic line parents are hearing in counseling is, 'Look, you want a live son or a dead daughter?'"[91]

Dr. Quentin Van Meter reiterates, "So the suicide is a myth. It's a total myth." He continues, "It's used as a hammer to guilt parents into doing this, and it's criminal."[92]

Dr. Susan Bradley reports that parents are put in a terrible position. "A lot of [parents] are faced with messages, some from the trans community, that if you don't accept your child [medically transitioning], they're going to go out and commit suicide." She adds, "And so you have to be accepting of them. And so they're caught between a rock and a hard place in terms of what, what do I really do now? Because I think this doesn't make sense, but I don't want my child to commit suicide."[93]

Of course this message is effective. A child's suicide is one of the worst things a parent could experience.

The 2020 documentary *Transforming Gender* illustrates the effectiveness of this emotional manipulation technique, as a father who transed his child asks, "Do I really want to see my kid attempt suicide?

No." Like so many other parents, this dad didn't even question the wisdom of transing his child.[94]

The mother of Max, a nine-year-old girl who is being transed, has completely bought into this lie as well. "This literally is a matter of life and death for so many young people who are dealing with these issues of identity, it's life or death, because the rate of suicide attempts in the trans community is 40% as families try to support their children and lessen the potential for self-harm."[95]

The reference Max's mother makes is most likely from the findings in the 2015 Transgender Survey published by the National Center for Transgender Equality. This survey is based on retrospective self-reports from a self-selected group identifying as transgender specifically recruited from trans activist organizations. The report states "Among the starkest findings is that 40% of respondents have attempted suicide in their lifetime—nearly nine times the attempted suicide rate in the US population (4.6%)."[96]

Kimberly Shappley admits she suspected that her son was gay but rather than accept her effeminate son, she transed him, telling others, "I am a mom of a little girl who has a 41% suicide rate."[97]

Activists like Shappley use the 40% cited in the 2015 Transgender Survey or the 41% pulled from *Injustice at Every Turn: A report of the National Transgender Discrimination Survey*, published by the national Center for Transgender Equality and the National Gay and Lesbian Task Force,[98] to claim that if children who have been transed don't get what they want (or in cases like Shappley's, what the parent wants), the child will attempt suicide.

But if these numbers are accurate, they actually suggest that transing dramatically *increases* the rates of suicide, a compelling argument against transitioning as a recommended treatment for gender dysphoria.

What these parents either haven't been told or don't understand, is that kids who are not transed don't actually have these high rates of suicide attempts or completed suicides. Children who do not transition are able to find ways to manage or resolve their difficult feelings.

Dr. Marcus Evans, who used to work at the Tavistock clinic in the U.K., said that there is a belief that transing kids is a "magical cure," when in fact these are kids who often are struggling with complex issues. Being told that transing will cure any suicidal ideation is not only wrong, but it is harmful to tell children that all their problems will instantly vanish upon transing.[99]

Lou, a detransitioner, said that she was never given another treatment option. Healthcare professionals told her that if she didn't transition, "'You will self-harm and you will kill yourself.' I became convinced that my options were transition or die."[100]

Luca, another detransitioner shared a similar story, "They told me that I have a gender dysphoria, and I said, 'Well, what is that?' And they explained it to me and, and I said, 'What are my options?' And they said, 'You can have sex change or you can commit suicide.'"[101]

Ethical doctors are working hard to dispel this dangerous suicide myth using credible research and reliable data.

Dr. Paul Hruz says, "The prevention of suicide is driving most of these recommendations. The claim is that if you do not participate in this care, your child will die by suicide. But when we look at the scientific evidence, it doesn't support that assertion."[102]

These claims of suicide are completely unsubstantiated, in fact the Senior Clinical Neuropsychologist for the state of Texas, Dr. Alan Hopewell testified in early 2021 that he was unable to document a single instance where a child completed a suicide as a result of not being given transing medical interventions.[103]

* * *

Shappley's suicide claim is nothing less than an attempt to manipulate school officials into allowing her son into the girl's bathroom.

We often hear from activists that since "41%" of those who have transed are suicidal, children should be transed. Or we hear that a "41%" attempted suicide rate proves that society should be coerced into using the pronouns and names of those who claim a transgender identity.

But the numbers don't in any way corroborate activists' claims.

If 41% of those who transition attempt suicide and the rate of completed suicides for those who medically transition is nineteen times higher than those who don't transition, the logical conclusion must be that transitioning dramatically increases both suicide attempts and completions.

Are there any other conditions, which can almost always be resolved on their own or with appropriate talk therapy, where healthcare providers intervene with a "treatment" that results in a dramatic increase in suicidality? Such a situation would be outrageous.

And yet, this is exactly what is happening.

Doctors and therapists are putting children on a treatment path of medicalization and increased rates of suicidality for a condition that is treatable with watchful waiting or talk therapy. Transition interventions damages children's bodies, cause lifelong complications, and profoundly increase their risk of death by suicide.

Unthinkable.

UCLA doctor Dr. Brandon Ito seems to understand this. "Approximately 40 to 50% of transgender adults [report] a prior suicide attempt in their life. When we compare this to the general US population statistic of less than 5%, we can see that this is definitely an increased and serious issue that we want to make sure to address."[104]

The outcomes for children currently being transed are likely to be even worse than they've been historically, because children today are taught that they can't handle difficult feelings and that transing will cure them. Children are lied to by the very people who should help them.

Dr. William Malone is incredulous as he watches vulnerable children being treated on the basis of an ideology rather than science. "The long-term studies show that in terms of psychological functioning, it doesn't help. It doesn't work. You know, suicidality actually increased."

Describing what should be obvious, Dr. Malone goes on to say, "You're supposed to do the experiments first to show that the treatment works, especially when you're talking about infertility and sexual dysfunction, long-term, and a four-fold, a four times increased risk of heart disease and a two to three times increased rate of development of blood clots and strokes. And the data we have now shows a twenty-fold increase risk of suicide long-term. So if we're going to go down that treatment protocol, there better be very good evidence that it works, and that evidence does not exist."

Such evidence does not exist.

Dr. Malone concludes, "This entire approach runs contrary to how we practice medicine in every other area."[105]

Addendum

The American Association of Suicidology, in collaboration with numerous other groups, has important recommendations for how the media should cover stories involving suicide, because studies have shown that suicide can be a social contagion. When children see reports of suicide, they are more likely to consider suicide an option. Studies have found that that suicide attempts go up when media coverage of suicide increases. Dramatic headlines and repeated coverage increase the rate of suicides, and the American Association of Suicidology cautions the media to be careful in how suicide is reported: "The way media cover suicide can influence behavior negatively by contributing to contagion or positively by encouraging help-seeking."[106]

When trans-rights activists insist that children will kill themselves if not granted everything they demand, activists generate a self-fulfilling prophesy; their rhetoric increases the likelihood that children will kill themselves.

The National Suicide Prevention Lifeline: 800-273-TALK (8255)

A SHORT HISTORY OF TRANSING

"Is there anything natural about stopping normal puberty? Would you stunt a child's normal eye development to make tiny eyes in an enlarging head? Would you stop a child's limb development so that the torso lengthens, but arms and legs remain stunted? This sounds bizarre, because it is. But it is analogous in many ways to the ongoing experiment in stopping normal puberty."

—Dr. Michael Laidlaw[107]

Dr. Quentin Van Meter refers to Alfred Kinsey, psychologist John Money, and Harry Benjamin as the "three musketeers." Most assume wrongly that the three were licensed medical doctors. Not one was.

Kinsey, Money, and Benjamin pioneered the idea of transsexualism, what would later become known as transgenderism, and they introduced the idea of gender identity as "the internal sexed self as either male or female."[108]

Harry Benjamin began medically transitioning adults in the 1950's. He provided medical services to Christine Jorgensen, one of the first men to be medically altered to appear more feminine.[109]

John Money embraced the idea of using medical interventions on those who experienced discomfort with their biological sex, and he had a clinic at Johns Hopkins in Baltimore. This clinic conducted a wide range of medical interventions, including cutting off healthy body parts in what was then called sex-change surgery.[110]

When the results of his interventions were finally examined, John Money was discredited. His clinic was shut down after a study by Jon Meyer showed that the surgeries provided "no objective advantage in terms of social rehabilitation."[111]

It wasn't until the mid-2000s when interest in altering the external appearance of those suffering from gender dysphoria experienced a resurgence. Transgender-rights activists began insisting that gender dysphoric children be treated with puberty blockers, cross-sex hormones, and even surgery.

This activism corresponded with increasing complaints about the serious side effects of Lupron, one of the most commonly prescribed puberty blockers.[112] A lawsuit in which men who took testosterone to improve their virility was settled around that time, and a study was published suggesting that hormone replacement therapy in menopausal women increased the risk of cancer.[113, 114]

Pharmaceutical companies seem to have wanted a new market for the puberty blockers and hormones that had previously garnered profits via adults. With the advent of the "trans kid" phenomenon, pharmaceutical companies suddenly had a market for all these drugs that were losing their consumer bases.

* * *

No research has been conducted to determine whether puberty blockers and cross-sex hormones are effective for the treatment of gender dysphoria. However, ample research shows they are instead quite harmful.[115, 116, 117, 118]

No research is needed to recognize that chopping off healthy body parts like breasts and testicles causes irreversible harm.[119] And despite activists' claims to the contrary, these unethical surgeries are happening regularly.

Girls as young as thirteen have their breasts sliced off.[120] Boys as young as sixteen have their testicles removed and their penis inverted to create a fake vaginal pouch.[121]

It is impossible to find out exactly how many children are on these damaging drugs and hormones, or how many have been mutilated by surgeries, because this information is not reported to any centralized body or even to local health departments. But the number of children being seen at gender clinics across the country is increasing at an astronomical rate.[122]

The one transing intervention that must be reported is prescriptions of the cross-sex hormone testosterone. Because testosterone is a powerful steroid it is on the controlled substance registry so health departments get information when it is prescribed.

In Utah five girls underwent a "medical transition" from female to male with the use of testosterone in 2015. By 2019 the number of girls prescribed testosterone exploded to 553.[123] Because estrogen is not a controlled substance, there is no way to know how many boys are being medically transitioned.

If the numbers are growing this fast in Utah, one of the most conservative states in the nation, they are likely growing at even more alarming rates in other states.

THE MYTH OF TRANSGENDERISM

"There is no one way that a woman thinks. Women are people. We are people like any man is a person. Our thoughts and interests and personalities are as varied and complex as any other person's. Testosterone withdrawal will make you miserable, but once it's over, if you're feeling better and you really don't want to go back on it, you probably aren't trans. It's crazy how deep internalized lesbophobia and misogyny can go. I always felt like 'one of the guys,' and was pissed that I wasn't treated like one. It didn't mean I was one — it meant I wanted to be treated like an equal. I wanted people to see me as someone who didn't think like a woman. But there is no one way a woman thinks. We are people.

"You can live in denial for years and years and years. You can convince yourself of anything to keep your head in the sand, and you may not have any idea that you're doing it. I know this because I did, and it took me years to realize. But the moment you accept that you don't have to be any way, that women AREN'T any way, that your dysphoria IS socialized, that you can live as whoever you want... It's extremely liberating. I have never known or been as happy with myself than I am now. Don't live a life you don't think you want just because you don't want people to be annoyed or think it's 'shitty' that you're going back. It is your life. It is your body. It is not a prison. If you make it one, you will never be happy."

—Posted by lez-dykawitz*

Those who advocate for administering puberty blockers to children, and who want to make it illegal for therapists to help children accept their bodies, do not want to hear stories like mine.

When I first started talking about my childhood "trans" identity, there were not very many people talking about their experience of identifying as transgender. But every day more voices share similar stories about suffering from gender dysphoria and not just surviving, but thriving without transitioning (or after detransitioning).

These are stories of people who have made peace with their bodies and with themselves. These stories demonstrate that watchful waiting or talk therapy to address underlying issues works. Such stories fly in the face of trans-rights activists' relentless claim that affirming gender dysphoric feelings is the only treatment for this complex mental health issue.

When I started to tell people about my childhood struggle with gender dysphoria, I got some interesting reactions.

Women who also suffered from gender dysphoria as children have reached out to me, to tell me they are living comfortably as women now that they are grown-ups. Both men and women relate to me how thankful they are that when they were growing up, children who didn't adhere to gender stereotypes were accepted, rather than labeled as gender non-conforming and transitioned.

Transgender-rights activists have dismissed me, wrongly declaring that I must have had a very mild form of gender dysphoria since I didn't assume a lifelong transgender identity.

I have heard from many gender dysphoric people who transitioned, thinking it would help, but who then found themselves physically damaged by and still suffering from invasive medical interventions.

And I have heard from a number of transgender-rights and social justice advocates who dismiss me as "transphobic," "homophobic," "misogynistic," and "bigoted."

* * *

Gender identity disorder and gender dysphoria in children has historically been extremely rare. However, the rate has increased rapidly as children who are too young to understand that their sex is immutable are being pressured to transition as early as toddlerhood.

Transgender activist Diane Ehrensaft even claims that when a male toddler unsnaps his onesie, he is making a "dress" in order to tell his parents he is actually a girl. Ehrensaft claims that if a baby girl pulls the barrettes from her hair, she is communicating that she is actually a boy born in the wrong body. Ehrensaft and other transgender-rights activists often speak about parents as if they are morons for not realizing they have "assigned" their baby the wrong sex.[124]

* * *

These toddlers and young children do not have gender dysphoria, but rather are children of parents who have embraced the idea that a girl who acts in stereotypically male ways is actually a boy stuck in a girl's body, and a boy who behaves in a stereotypically feminine manner is actually girl stuck in a boy's body.

These children are too young to make even the most basic decisions about their lives. In some cases are not even potty trained, and yet parents are transing them to make them appear as the opposite sex.

Pushing transition on children isn't always the parents' fault, however. Transgender-rights activists have done a breathtakingly thorough job convincing society that children are likely to kill themselves if they are not allowed to transition. They argue that the younger a "trans" child transitions, the better off the child will be.

Transgender-rights activists have convinced parents that providing therapy to children who actually are suffering gender dysphoria is abusive.

Transgender-rights activists insist that being transgender is not a mental illness and should not be treated as one.

Transgender-rights activists have lobbied doctors to endorse managing gender dysphoria with puberty blockers in children as young as eight years old.

Transgender-rights activists have suggested that once a child is on puberty blockers for a couple of years, the child should be given cross-hormones.

Transgender-rights activists push teens to undergo mutilating surgeries. Don't believe this happens? Dr. Johanna Olsen-Kennedy, a recipient of a National Institute of Health grant reported that she prescribes puberty blockers and cross-sex hormones to eight-year-old children.[125]

The message from transgender-rights activists is that children who are gender non-conforming will be happier and healthier as adults if they transition as children, forgo normal puberty, take hormones to force their body to develop sex characteristics of the opposite sex, and finally undergo invasive surgical procedures that eliminate sex organs of the opposite sex, and confer fake sex organs of the opposite gender.

How can anything about that pathway lead to better outcomes than simply helping a gender dysphoric child to learn to accept and love his or her own natural, healthy body?

Transgender-rights activists are ecstatic about welcoming these young "members" to the transgender community. Pharmaceutical companies are equally ecstatic about new lifelong customers of expensive cross-sex hormones.

So transgender-rights activists and pharmaceutical companies don't want to admit that people like me exist, because we are living, breathing contradictions to their narrative.

But we do exist, and in ever larger numbers as more and more early adopters of this nefarious ideology wake up and realize what a lie they believed. We are a testament to the fact that children with gender dysphoria don't have to transition. We are evidence that less invasive and ultimately more successful approaches to helping children with gender dysphoria exist.

Transgender-rights activists make a lot of claims about the biological basis of gender dysphoria, but in reality no evidence exists to support the concept that male- and female-gendered souls can be born in the wrong body.

Although I tend to act in ways that might be described as "masculine," biological fact makes it clear that I am female. Was I born with the personality and preferences I have, or did my personality and preferences change as a result of my experiences and environment? Probably, like everything related to human development, the answer is a little of both.

After I was sexually assaulted, I decided I was a boy. I got in trouble in first grade for being too aggressive both verbally and physically. But I was willing to be completely socially ostracized in order to protect myself from being sexually violated again. I did everything I could to act like a boy. When I could get away with it, I even used the boys' bathroom instead of the girls'. In my little girl mind, I was sure that if I made my mind up to be a boy, at some point the rest of the world would forget that I was a girl and accept me as a boy.

And then I would be safe.

I hated it when I had to dress up as a girl. When I had to wear a dress, I was afraid. I felt vulnerable.

In grade school, I played by myself at recess. I stayed away from the girls because I didn't want to be associated with them. But I didn't play with the boys, either. They chased me away and told me I couldn't play.

When I was required to play with girls during gym class, they would often run crying to the teacher, saying that I was mean. I did not play like the other girls who were doing cartwheels and whispering to each other.

By the time I was in fifth grade, I had a nickname, "Erin Underarm Strong," because I often challenged boys to arm wrestling, to show that I was as tough as they were. Despite my small size, I often won, even when I was up against bigger, older boys.

That nickname was a way for kids to make fun of me, both for my arm wrestling, as well as for my poor hygiene.

* * *

Despite what some would consider my many male characteristics, I am female, without question. This doesn't mean I "identify" as female, it means I *am* female.

I have never "identified" as female; I don't even know what it means. Nor do any of the women I talk to. We all shake our heads with incredulity wondering what it must be like for men who claim to believe they feel like women.

What is the essence of woman, so elusive and indefinable to me and my female friends, to which these men lay claim?

* * *

Though it took until my early twenties to start appreciating my body, I finally achieved it when I had children. Having my babies allowed me to appreciate my female body in a way that is difficult to describe. I felt in awe of my body's ability to gestate a baby, give birth, and then nurse my children. Maternal instincts were unleashed in me that I hadn't known existed, or that I was capable of feeling.

I am not suggesting that having a baby cures gender dysphoria, but rather that having a baby allowed me to connect with my female body in a way that I wasn't able to before.

To be honest, even now after all these years, I still have twinges of gender dysphoria.

They don't come because I am stuck in the wrong body, but because sometimes my thinking goes a bit off. When I am stressed or in a difficult situation, my default response is often, "I'd be better off if I were a man," or "I hate being a woman," or "Why am I stuck in this body?"

These are old messages which started after I was sexually assaulted, and they've stuck with me throughout my life. We all have these kinds of unhelpful self-messages that we pick up as children. Just as the survivor of anorexia nervosa is inclined to think she is fat when her life starts feeling out of control, or as someone struggling with OCD is compelled to wash his hands when he feels stressed, the default response to difficulty for someone who suffers from gender dysphoria will be a feeling that they'd be better off as the opposite sex.

But there are good techniques such as cognitive behavioral therapy that can help anyone who suffers from difficult feelings. Changing one's body is not a real solution.[126]

* * *

Were I a kid today, I would almost certain be put on puberty blockers. The therapist or doctor would start me on wrong-sex hormones soon after, and I would eventually have my breasts lopped off.

I also suspect I would have killed myself, because my dysphoria was a mental disorder that would not have been cured by mutilating my body. In fact, changing my body so significantly would have deprived me the opportunity to make peace with it. I also would have been deprived the chance to process the underlying issues that caused me to have such hatred for myself as a female. Attempting to transition also would have affirmed my delusion that I was better off being a man than a woman.

Those of us who have experienced gender dysphoria serious enough to cause general dysfunction are not giddy with excitement about transitioning, we just want relief from our difficult feelings; similarly, people who feel suicidal don't typically want to die, they just can't see any other way to make the pain stop.

For "experts" to insist that the only way to address gender dysphoria is to damage a healthy body is beyond unethical.

* * *

My dysphoria was a reaction to my sexual assault, and was intensified by my mother telling me that my father wanted a boy instead of a girl. The dysphoria was continually reinforced as I saw my brother benefiting from being a boy and from me being treated badly for not conforming to traditional gender stereotypes.

The discomfort those of us with gender dysphoria experience is not because anything is wrong with our bodies. The pain isn't cured by hormones or surgery or different clothing or makeup. These are just superficial attempts to cover up the dysphoria. These interventions may temporarily distract us from the dysphoria, but they are neither healthy nor lasting ways to manage or resolve the problem.

Transgender-rights activists put pressure on the American Psychiatric Association to change the diagnosis of "gender identity disorder" to "gender dysphoria." This change was made in the *Diagnostic and Statistical Manual, Fifth Edition* (DSM-5) to "remove the stigma" of transgenderism being considered a mental disorder.[127]

Increasingly, the term "gender dysphoria" is used to describe emotional distress felt because of how society reacts to those who believe they have a mismatch between biological sex and gender identity. This change in diagnosis has allowed transgender-rights activists to discredit therapeutic approaches for treating gender dysphoria. They insist that transitioning is the only appropriate response to gender dysphoria, because the dysphoria isn't a mental disorder but an inherent flaw.

In other words, the American Psychiatric Association uses traditional stereotypical gender behavior to diagnose gender dysphoria. Failing to adhere to gender norms is enough to get a diagnosis of gender dysphoria.

Since transgender-rights activists push those with gender dysphoria to transition, it means that anyone who is gender non-conforming is encouraged to transition. Rather than removing the stigma of having a mental disorder, this approach has pathologized gender non-conformity.

* * *

Insisting that a child who is gender non-conforming is transgender reinforces traditional gender stereotypes.

The American Psychiatric Association has swallowed transgender-rights activists' worldview hook, line, and sinker. The first item they list for giving a diagnosis of gender dysphoria in a child is, "a marked incongruence between one's experienced/expressed gender and assigned gender."[128]

Children's gender is not assigned. A child is born male or female, and that binary difference is observed, not assigned.

To call gender "assigned" encourages the misconception that someone can be born into the wrong body. Activists who propagate this lie assert that a lack of conformity to gender stereotypes is not an appropriate expression of the ways in which males and females express themselves, but rather an indication of a biological disconnect between sex and gender. Shockingly, this incongruence between sex and gender experience or expression only has to last a few months in order for activists to proclaim a child transgender.

Anyone who has worked around children knows that children regularly insist that they are something they are not. In fact, children try on different identities in an effort to explore the world, which is why children engage in make-believe play.

The DSM-5 actually lists one of the diagnostic criteria as, "In boys, a strong rejection of typically masculine toys, games, and activities and a strong avoidance of rough-and-tumble play; or in girls a strong rejection of typically feminine toys, games, and activities."

Why is the DSM-5 forcing regressive sex stereotypes on children?

* * *

Both the American Psychiatric Association and the World Professional Association on Transgender Health admit that most gender dysphoria does not persist into adulthood. So why do therapists and medical providers pressure children to transition anyway?[129, 130]

One of the things that helped me overcome my gender dysphoria was recognizing that traditional gender stereotypes do not define me as a female. Just because I have more masculine behaviors and characteristics does not mean that I am a man; it means I am a woman who is not conforming to traditional gender stereotypes.

When I struggle with dysphoria now, I move my thoughts toward all the things my body allows me to do. It can enjoy chocolate, feel the warmth of sun on a cool winter day, play in the rain, pet my cat, and walk in the woods. All of these things I can do because of my body. I remember to be consciously grateful for my body and to remember that my body and I are one.

I remind myself that the feelings of disconnect I have with my body aren't my body's fault, but are the result of trauma and harmful stereotypes about how my body is supposed to look and how I am supposed to act.

It infuriates me when people reinforce harmful gender stereotypes by encouraging children who deviate from the norm to believe they are in the wrong body. "Male" or "female" toys, clothing, and activities do not exist. The entire definition of gender dysphoria is subservient to sexist gender roles.

One of the reasons that children are not conforming to traditional gender roles is that society has (rightly and helpfully) agreed that imposing these traditional roles limits both males and females. But today transgender-rights activists tell children that if they don't conform to traditional gender roles, something is inherently wrong with them.

Activists tell children that if they don't conform to traditional gender roles, it is because they were born in the wrong body. That is nothing but a heinous lie.

* * *

Because of previous medical abuses of children and the mentally ill, children and/or people who suffer with mental illness are considered a protected category by medical providers and unable to give legal consent for medical interventions, especially interventions that will cause life-long damage to their otherwise healthy body.[131]

Transgender-rights activists claim that children—even children who suffer with disorders such as autism, OCD, depression, *etc.*—are capable of consenting to life-altering treatments that promote disassociation from their own bodies, damage healthy organs and systems, and lead to worsened physical and psychological outcomes.

By aligning ourselves with trans-rights activists' demands, we affirm the acceptance of a harmful delusion, rather than encouraging children with dysphoria to work toward accepting and loving themselves. Furthermore, we are lying to children when we allow transgender-rights activists to tell children that boys can have vaginas and girls can have penises.

I am thankful that I had supportive teachers and counselors who guided my obsessive focus on my body outward towards more healthy activities, rather than pushed me toward greater delusion and self-harm, as is the practice today.

* * *

I am thankful for therapists who taught me how to challenge my internal monologue of constant criticism, and I want today's children to receive the same appropriate psychological care.

I am grateful for therapists who helped me understand that my gender dysphoria was a coping mechanism my creative mind came up with to help me make sense of my trauma, and I want today's children to have the benefit of trustworthy and ethical therapists who won't push them into medical transition.

I am thankful to all the people who helped me realize that a female can express her gender in non-stereotypical ways and that is okay, and I want today's children to learn the same powerful lessons.

I want today's children to be safe and healthy instead of damaged by transing.

WHAT DOES THE RESEARCH SAY?

"The child and the parents are being encouraged to believe that if they take the next step, the anxiety and the sorrow and the woundedness will go away. So they start with puberty blockade and transitioning. There's a lot of excitement, but you haven't addressed the problems. So, it's time to go to the next step. We're going to go to cross-sex hormones. You get somebody cross sex-hormones, they'll feel like a giant for a while and you will think, 'Oh, I've done them a great good.' It's a passing thing. And so the anxiety is still there and then they'll progress, so really what we need to do next is surgery and it's just because the interior wound has not been addressed."

—Dr. Patrick Lappert[132]

Though transgender-rights activists assert that research undergirds the transing of children, none actually does. No sound research supports transitioning sexes to cure gender dysphoria, nor does any data suggest that transitioning reduces the distress of gender dysphoria better than therapeutic treatments such as cognitive behavioral therapy, or even doing nothing at all.

No research exists regarding the long-term consequences of medically transing children, because this "treatment path" is such a new phenomenon. The research we do have, which looks at adults who medically transition, finds that no benefit exists to medically transitioning with respect to improved psychiatric outcomes. In fact, considerable drawbacks are prevalent.

Swedish pro-transgender researcher Richard Bränström, who says he has an "intersectional perspective," and his colleague, John Pachankis, revealed that mental health outcomes for those who medically transition are worse than those who don't transition. The participants in the study who surgically transitioned had higher levels of psychiatric medications prescribed, an increase in psychiatric visits, and a higher rate of hospitalizations following suicide attempts.[133]

Another of the very few longitudinal studies which exist followed the progress of all citizens in Sweden who medically transitioned, and found that those who underwent surgery experienced considerably higher risks for mortality, suicidal behavior, and psychiatric morbidity than the general population. This population's completed suicide rate proved an astonishing nineteen and a half times *higher* than the general population.

In addition, these researchers found, "Sex-reassigned persons had a higher risk of inpatient care for a psychiatric disorder other than gender identity disorder than controls matched on birth year and birth sex." The same study reported, "The most striking result was the high mortality rate in both male-to-females and female-to males, compared to the general population."

The study's author concludes, "This highlights that post-surgical transsexuals are a risk group that need long-term psychiatric and somatic follow-up. Even though surgery and hormonal therapy alleviates gender dysphoria, it is apparently not sufficient to remedy the high rates of morbidity and mortality found among transsexual persons."[134]

Again, as in the Bränström and Pachankis study, these researchers held a perspective that transing was an appropriate treatment for gender dysphoria. But the research flies in the face of those who insist that transing is a cure for gender dysphoria, or even a good way of managing it.

The research shows clearly that transing kids puts them on a dangerous and difficult path that will leave them at higher risk for poor outcomes.

Dr. Kenneth Zucker's career-long research found that the gender dysphoria is very often resolved naturally. Dr. Zucker advocated a watchful waiting approach for children with gender dysphoria, because most children's gender dysphoria resolves during puberty.

This is a far better outcome than that experienced by those who are transed.

Dr. Zucker and his research team's most recent longitudinal study on boys with gender dysphoria found an astonishing rate of 87.8% desistance in gender dysphoria. In other words these boys were not just managing their gender dysphoria, but their gender dysphoria actually resolved without any need for invasive medical interventions.[135]

Dr. Lisa Littman says in the *National Review* that, "Activists appear to follow a very conscious strategy of harassment and intimidation, which I'm sure they feel is justified. They go after the reputations of the people they wish to silence, and they also attack the organizations those people are affiliated with, offering to back off if only those organizations take swift and decisive disciplinary action. The decision to make a medical transition is a difficult one and people need accurate information about risks, benefits and alternatives to assess whether, in their individual case, it will be beneficial — that is the essence of informed consent. When activists shut down gender dysphoria research about potential risks and contraindications of transition, they are depriving the transgender community of their right to receive accurate information."[136]

If solid, evidence-based research existed to support transing kids, why would researchers be bullied at all? Why don't we see vigorous debate around this issue?

Because trans-rights activists want to transition children based on their belief system, not based upon science. Their beliefs are centered on the concept of a gendered soul that is somehow put into the wrong body prior to birth; this ideology originates from mysticism, not from evidence-based research.

* * *

Susan Bewley, Professor Emeritus Obstetrics & Women's Health, writes in her article *Safeguarding Adolescents from Premature, Permanent Medicalization*, "While respecting individuals' right to a different viewpoint, it is neither mandatory to affirm their beliefs nor automatic that transition is the goal, particularly when dealing with children, adolescents and young adults. These risk closing the 'open future', as well as life-long physical problems including lack of sexual function, infertility and medical dependency. With 85% desistance amongst referred transgender children and increasing awareness of detransitioning, unquestioning 'affirmation' as a pathway that leads gender dysphoric patients to irreversible interventions cannot be considered sole or best practice."[137]

In *The Sunday Times*, Andrew Gilligan reports that, "England's only NHS gender clinic for children is exposing young patients to 'long-term damage' because of its 'inability to stand up to the pressure' from 'highly politicized' campaigners and families demanding fast-track gender transition, some of its own doctors say."[138]

A report compiled by former staff governor at the Tavistock clinic in the UK, Dr. David Bell notes, "some children 'take up a trans identity as a solution' to 'multiple problems such as historic child abuse in the family, bereavement . . . homophobia and a very significant incidence of autism spectrum disorder' after being 'coached' online and by trans activist groups."

He goes on to report that staff at the clinic had "huge and unmanageable caseloads" and were afraid of being accused of transphobia if they questioned a child's desire to transition."[139]

In a recent court ruling, the UK High Court admitted that these interventions are experimental and not medically sound.[140]

When doctors are bullied if they do not accept a belief system not grounded in science or data, the situation sounds a lot more like cult indoctrination than application of appropriate standards of care.

* * *

How did these interventions become the medically "accepted" standard of care?

In the case of transgender medical interventions, it started with WPATH, the World Professional Association of Transgender Health, originally formed by Harry Benjamin, who exhibited a predilection for experimenting on children.[141, 142]

WPATH's purpose is to advocate for transgenderism. This organization developed the first pathway for medical transition. The WPATH guidelines were pushed into other professional organizations under the guise of being "tolerant and inclusive," without any actual evidence to support the guidelines' use.

And, despite WPATH's insistence on following so-called "standards of care," gender clinics flagrantly disregard the very standards to which they claim to adhere. For example, WPATH has cautioned that most children with gender dysphoria do not grow up to be transgender if not told they are transgender and encouraged to transition. WPATH suggests that children be at least sixteen before being prescribed cross-sex hormones as a treatment for gender dysphoria, and they recommend that no children have cosmetic surgery to change their external appearance. These surgeries should wait until the child is an adult, according to WPATH.

However, we see clinics transing young children via experimental medical interventions at increasingly younger ages. Doctors at gender clinics give children as young as eight years old cross-sex hormones, and remove the breasts from girls as young as thirteen years old.[143, 144, 145]

Activist groups such as The Trevor Project and the Human Rights Campaign have systematically eradicated the tried-and-true treatment option of watchful waiting and talk therapy, denigrating such appropriate and effective care as "conversion therapy." In their efforts to ban ethical care by conflating it with unethical and abusive practices that were formerly used in attempts to change gay people's same-sex attractions, trans-rights activists have actually instituted a heinous conversion therapy protocol which denies vulnerable children access to the mental health services that would help them process the underlying issues causing their dysphoria.

Trans-rights activists fraudulently insist that affirming a child's gender dysphoria is the only treatment. Again, this course of treatment is akin to a doctor agreeing that a severely underweight anorexic is indeed fat and should get liposuction and gastric surgery. Gender "affirmation" is no different from affirming someone's paranoid delusions that people actually are out to get him and he should hide in his closet. Confirming attempted gender transition is just like telling a depressed child who cuts herself that cutting is appropriate, and then giving her a better razor blade with which to do it.

When it comes to transing kids, not only are health care providers affirming a child's belief that they are inherently flawed, the doctors are providing medicalized self-harm to a distressed child and denying the child the opportunity to actually heal.

* * *

In a 2021 review of the quality of guidelines for transing gender dysphoric people, even researchers who support transgender ideology found that "topics are linked to a weak evidence base, with variations in methodological rigor and lack of stakeholder involvement." They also found that the quality of the best available evidence in support of transing anyone (let alone children) was "poor."[146]

When those who are supportive of the concept that people can be born in the wrong body admit that the so-called "standards of care" are based on poor quality evidence, and that those who are being transed are not provided accurate and honest information about the pros and cons of transing, it is clear that this approach is problematic.

In summary, the longitudinal research shows that transing kids is likely to result in poor outcomes. The evidence to support the transing of kids is either completely lacking or of poor quality. But most significantly, transing kids does not cure gender dysphoria.[147]

We know that most kids will outgrow their gender dysphoria. We know that transing kids causes incredible damage to children's bodies. The research and evidence are clear. Transing kids is, as pediatrician Dr. Michelle Cretella says, "a massive social and medical experiment that is completely unregulated and it's also not fully consented."[148]

THERAPY BANS

"I think we as detrans people have to start forcing our way into the conversation. If someone is thinking about transitioning they should have all the information they can. I can't believe how the medical community has just signed off on this. Especially the mental health community. Unfortunately if a therapist so much as brings up that maybe transition isn't the only option they risk losing their license."

—Posted by ajf2077*

"Yes the conversion therapy law in California includes transgender people, which is frickin' insane. It will cause great harm. No matter where you go for therapy in California, the minute you say you are trans, the only thing the therapist can do is agree with you."

—Posted by bkp13*

In 2019, Equality Utah (a pro-LGBT rights organization) sent me a letter asking me to help them raise funds to support the passage of the "Ethical Therapy for Minors Act." What an innocuous sounding bit of legislation. Who wouldn't support ethical therapy for our kids?

When I investigated, I found out the bill aimed to prohibit any kind of "conversion" therapy.

Horror stories have circulated about gays and lesbians being given electric shocks, or told that their families or God will not love them unless they become heterosexual. There have even been stories of lesbians being gang raped to "cure" them from same sex attraction. This is what most people think of when they hear the term "conversion therapy."

But those horrific abuses are no longer what's meant by the term "conversion therapy," as used by transgender-rights activists. The misleading attempts in Utah and elsewhere to ban any therapy other than "affirming" a child's "trans" identity, prevents therapists from doing anything except encouraging children to dissociate from themselves and to medicalize their bodies. Therapists are now prevented from helping children actually cope with and heal from gender dysphoric feelings.

In states that have these bans, parents who question whether their child is suffering from something other than a transgender identity are told by healthcare professionals that it is unethical for a therapist to challenge the child's identity. These bans brand a child's so-called "identity" as sacrosanct. By deeming it unethical for therapists to challenge a child's identity, these bans imply that it is also unethical for society or even parents to challenge a child's identity.

Currently the United Nations is working to ban "conversion therapy" worldwide. This international effort would make it illegal for not just healthcare providers but for any adult—including parents—to do anything other than affirm a child's gender dysphoric feelings and move the child onto a path of medicalization.

Conversion therapy bans are not about the ethical treatment of children. They are politically and financially motivated strategies to line the pockets of the gender clinicians, pharmaceutical companies, and cosmetic surgeons.

The request for a donation from Equality Utah ended by saying, "And while legislation alone can't heal every wound, it will ensure that the next generations never endure these humiliating and dangerous practices. To reduce the rates of suicide we must send a message to every LGBTQ child: you belong, you are loved and your life has value — just as you are."[149]

In other words, if you don't support us, you are responsible for the suicide of LGBTQ children. This rhetoric is not only ridiculous, it is treacherous.

I posted my concerns to Equality Utah's Facebook page, and asked them to send me the exact wording of the act they were planning on introducing, but instead of responding, they deleted my comments and blocked me.

Though I knew I was risking a lot by speaking against their bill, for the first time in my life I testified before a legislative hearing.

Taking a stand against Equality Utah cost me a lot. I lost friends and family. I jeopardized my career. I exposed something deeply personal about myself for public scrutiny. But I felt ethically compelled to stand up for the rights of children who, like me, suffer from gender dysphoria. Children with gender dysphoria need real support and appropriate mental health services in order to manage and resolve their dysphoria.

Though Equality Utah was unsuccessful in passing their legislation, shortly after the legislative session with pressure from activists, the Utah Division of Occupational and Professional Licensing passed a rule banning health care providers who have professional licenses in Utah from helping children understand the underlying causes of their gender dysphoria. The conversion therapy ban got slipped in the back door.

* * *

Transgender-rights activists promote therapy bans via misleading scare tactics based on false information.

By hitching their wagon to the LGB, the T created a compelling narrative. The so-called "research" used to push their agenda came from studies involving unscrupulous reparative therapy (which is already prohibited by the American Psychological Association) to change the attractions of gays and lesbians, and which has nothing to do with children suffering from gender dysphoria.

Therapy bans prevent access to appropriate mental healthcare services for children who developed gender dysphoria as a result of an underlying mental health issue. These bans also reinforce regressive sex stereotypes upon which the diagnosis of gender dysphoria is based in the first place.

No justification exists for denying children with gender dysphoria an opportunity to manage and resolve their feelings of distress via long-accepted and appropriate counseling techniques such as talk therapy.

Transgender-rights activists pejoratively refer to anyone who manages or resolved gender dysphoria as "converted." These activists don't want the healthiest outcomes for those suffering from gender dysphoria; they want to capture as many people into the transgender community as possible, for politics and profit. Transgender-rights activists further deny the existence of detransitioners' experiences when they convince parents to transition a gender-confused child by hiding the fact that a growing number of people wish desperately that they'd never attempted to transition in the first place.

Thankfully, those who realized the harm caused from being transed are starting to speak out.

Detransitioner Keira Bell, who won a lawsuit against the clinic that transed her as a child, said, "You feel so trapped and alone." She goes on to say, "it's so experimental because, you know, doctors don't even know, you know, the outcomes of a lot of these treatments that are given out."[150]

Cole had her breasts removed at sixteen and now regrets it, saying "I honestly don't think I was at an age when I was able to fully, like truly understand, take in all the different aspects of that."[151]

Even pro-transing doctor and the director of the Lurie Children's Hospital gender clinic Dr. Robert Garofalo recognizes that he and his colleagues are engaging in medical experimentation on children. He unabashedly says, "There just isn't a lot of evidence-based medicine to support the interventions that we're offering these families."[152]

A survey about detransitioning found that "the two most common reasons for detransition were shifting political/ideological beliefs (at almost 63%) and finding alternative coping mechanisms for dysphoria (59%)."[153]

These results are important because they suggest that a sizeable number of people transitioned not necessarily to manage gender dysphoria, but as a result of a political or ideological belief. This is consistent with comments detransitioners make, who often feel like they were coerced into transitioning.

Transgender-rights activists don't have clear criteria based on research for when a child is likely to persist with gender dysphoria into adulthood, nor do they have any research to inform a gender dysphoric profile that is not going to be responsive to other methods of treatment.

If transitioning were innocuous and reversible, then offering a trial transition might be acceptable. But attempting to medically transition sexes is neither innocuous nor fully reversible. Transing a child says to that child, "Something is inherently wrong with you—so wrong that we must retard your development, administer drugs to alter your external appearance, chop off your healthy body parts, and try to turn you into someone else."

MEDICALIZING GENDER DYSPHORIA

"I think a few things we have to take into account are

1. Young people do not have fully developed frontal lobes, which SERIOUSLY impacts decision making and future planning skills. Young people are more likely to be impulsive and overwhelmed by emotions, as they have neither the biological capability to think objectively about decision making nor the life experience to develop skills associated with emotional regulation and decision making. I didn't take this seriously before, but oh boy now I do.
2. Gender ideology is very popular among younger people in a way it isn't in older generations. As someone who began identifying as trans at 15 after finding it online, I believe this is largely a result of the things I described above.

"When you have more young people transitioning, you have more young people detransitioning. It's less that transitioning at a younger age poses more risk for detransition, and more about the age demographics that are transitioning in the first place. Many people are transitioning as soon as they turn 18 after identifying as trans throughout their teens, and detransitioning 2–5 years later. This is simply a larger group than the adults, because young people are more susceptible to ways of thinking that lead to making inappropriate decisions, especially since the trans movement 'affirms' their thoughts so strongly. Adults are more often equipped with life experience and cognitive skills that would allow them to think more critically about ideologies and personal decisions, so they are less likely to transition for the same reasons as we see in young people today. Obviously, older people who detransition very much exist and feel equally harmed by their experiences though. It's just that young brains are far more likely to fall down this rabbit hole, and brains that are more developed and equipped with lessons learned through living life are less likely to do the same as they would have been had they found transgenderism at a younger age."

—Posted by lacroicsz5*

As with most mental health conditions, many approaches to managing gender dysphoria exist.

It was generally expected that children, teens, and even adults went through periods of struggling with their body image. In fact, it was "normal" not to be 100% comfortable within oneself and no expectation existed that becoming completely comfortable with oneself was the goal. Rather, people understood that some discomfort was not just normal but even beneficial. If we always felt perfectly comfortable with ourselves, we would not experience the cues necessary to make sure we take care of ourselves, eat well, exercise, and sleep enough.

Some people are born with Congenital Insensitivity to Pain & Anhydrosis, a rare disease that leaves them without the ability to detect physical pain. They tend to die young because they don't have the protective impulses that keep them safe.

The same is true with psychological distress, which is the mind's way of letting us know that we need to address something.

In my case, my teacher and other adults recognized my distress. Today they would likely call my behavior "acting out," but back then the teacher just knew something wasn't right with me. My explanation for my behavior was "I am a boy," but my teacher knew better. She knew that a happy, well-adjusted girl doesn't suddenly become a boy who exhibits disturbing social behaviors. In fact, she knew that girls can't become boys.

My teacher got me help from the school psychologist and then, over the years, I worked with other mental healthcare professionals to process the trauma I had experienced.

Had I been transed, I would have been denied the opportunity to process my trauma, and the shame and self-hatred I had as a result of the sexual assault would only have been reinforced.

Had I been transed, I would have engaged in medicalized self-harm with irreversible interventions and lifelong medicalization, and I would never have experienced the joy of motherhood.

Furthermore, had I been transed, I would have found myself in situations where I could easily have been re-traumatized by another assault. I shudder when I think of little girls with gender dysphoria going into men's bathrooms and locker rooms.

Children have a hard time reporting sexual assault. They often believe the assault was somehow their fault, they worry they will not be believed, sometimes they are threatened by the assailant, and they worry they will get in trouble. Imagine how much harder it would be for a girl who is being "affirmed" as a boy to report? She would not want to admit an assault that confirmed that she is still a female, despite her best efforts to prove otherwise. She might have an increased sense that the assault was her fault if the assault occurred in the boys' locker room that she insisted she be allowed to use, or a men's bathroom that she used in an attempt to feel more masculine.

How have we gone from helping children process and manage underlying issues that cause discomfort to encouraging children to disassociate from themselves and assume a new identity?

Transgender-rights activists adopted and propagated a philosophy regarding the treatment of gender identity issues: they decided that people with gender dysphoria, or any feelings of discomfort with or about their sex or body, should be transitioned first socially and then medically.

On the surface that plan might seem to make sense.

If a girl doesn't like to wear dresses, let her wear pants. If a boy likes to play with dolls, buy him a Barbie. But this isn't about encouraging a child to dress for comfort or play with preferred toys; this is about telling a child that if s/he doesn't adhere to regressive gender stereotypes then s/he was born in the wrong body.

Social transition is all about adopting the stereotypical behavior of the opposite sex.

Girls who are uncomfortable being girls will get a haircut, wear superhero t-shirts, and change their names from Margaret to Max. Boys will grow their hair out, wear dresses—the more frills the better—and change their names from James to Juno.

Activists insist that it is critical for everyone who interacts with the child to use the child's "new" name and pronouns, and that the child be allowed to use the bathroom and locker room reserved for the opposite sex, and (if the child is athletic) to compete as the opposite sex.

The message these children hear is that all the adults around them believe that they are inherently flawed, that some terrible mistake was made and they got the wrong gender spirit for the body they occupy.

It isn't clear how the gender spirit supposedly enters the body or where it comes from, but the children are told by teachers, doctors, and therapists that a mismatch occurred and the only way to deal with the incongruity is to change their bodies to match their gender spirits.

As absurd as this ideology sounds (and is), social and medical transition is now the accepted "standard of care" that is damaging far too many children.

* * *

Activists deny that therapy is helpful in managing and resolving gender dysphoria, and they assert, without any proof, that therapy is harmful. No evidence exists to support transgender advocates' contention that transitioning is beneficial in any way, but much evidence indicates that transitioning can be extremely harmful to children.[154]

To complicate matters, people with mental health issues are, by definition, often unable to discern what is the appropriate treatment for them. This is especially the case for children with mental health issues.

Often people with mental health issues do not think clearly enough to understand that they have a mental illness. One of the biggest challenges mental healthcare providers face is something called *anosognosia*, which describes someone who rejects a diagnosis of mental illness. Anosognosia is common in individuals with dysphoria, dysmorphia, and other conditions in which an individual is hyper-focused on themselves.

Effective therapeutic treatments for gender dysphoria do exist. Unfortunately, transgender-rights activists have caused social anosognosia by insisting that gender dysphoria does not exist, but is instead evidence of transgenderism.

Our entire society has been told that we are hateful and bigoted if we do not accept these activists' worldview, which is a belief system that puts children and young adults on a pathway to lifelong medicalization. Anyone who points out that gender dysphoria is a mental health issue is called transphobic and vilified by transgender-rights activists.

We are not helping those with gender dysphoria by affirming their delusions; in fact, we are affirming their anosognosia. It is impossible to provide appropriate mental health services if transgender-rights activists are enabling their delusion that a "trans man" is a man and a "trans woman" is a woman.

Even if a distinct male gender or a distinct female gender could inhabit the body of a person of the opposite sex, medically transitioning children with puberty blockers that retard their development, cross-sex hormones that damage their bodies, and elective cosmetic surgery would still be unethical and unnecessary.

If a penis does not make a man male, then getting rid of it would not make a man female. If breasts do not make a woman female, then having breasts would not make a man female. If feminine physical characteristics do not make a woman female, then taking hormones to make a male body more look more female does not make a man female. If our bodies do not define our gender or sex, then a boy who is trapped in a girl's body needn't change that body, because the body would not define sex or gender.

And yet, transgender-rights activists hypocritically continue to push medical transition.

* * *

Research shows that gender identity and gender expression are malleable, and that oftentimes gender dysphoria is the result of underlying mental health struggles. The whole concept of gender fluidity is at direct odds with the idea that gender is fixed and that someone can be born in the wrong body. If gender is fluid it can't be fixed. If someone can come to the realization that they are the opposite gender at any point in their lives then gender is fluid.[155]

* * *

With respect to most (if not all) other mental health issues affecting children, parents are given a range of treatment options. The best treatment is usually considered to be the least invasive option with the fewest side effects and expectation of the best outcomes. Transing, with all it involves, is profoundly invasive, as it not only requires the child to change who they are, but requires everyone around the child to actively participate in the farce.

Children who are not old enough to vote, drive, rent a car, or sign for a student loan are dictating their medical care under the encouragement of activists who give them the false hope that transitioning will cure them of all their discomforts and distress.

HARMS OF MEDICAL TRANSITIONING

"I made the decision to begin detransition a month ago and since then I have felt like I am slowing waking up from some kind of weird alternate reality. How did I ever believe the things I did about trans issues or transition. I honestly feel like my brain was fucked with and it's incredibly depressing. I once thought that kids transitioning was totally fine. I now can't even fathom how we as a society are ok with this."

—Posted by ajf2077*

The age of eighteen years is recognized by researchers as the point at which a child becomes emotionally mature enough to agree to participate in a research study as a human subject. Prior to eighteen years of age, a child's legal parent or guardian has to consent for the child to be a human subject in a research study. Eighteen has been generally recognized as the age at which an individual can accept or refuse medical treatment. Those under eighteen can't typically even sign for a loan or rent a car, and young people can't legally purchase alcohol until twenty-one years of age.

As a society we have established eighteen the age of majority because we recognize that children's brains are not fully developed. They lack the capacity to make good long-term decisions. They tend to have difficulty with cost-benefit analysis and understanding risk.

* * *

I probably thought more about consent when I was a child than most children do.

Somewhere between the age of thirteen and fourteen, I fell in love with a friend of the family. Sometime after I turned fourteen, he claimed he had feelings for me as well. I will never forget the first time he pulled me toward him for a kiss: it was as if the world disappeared and he was the only thing that mattered.

He led me into his bedroom and I willingly went.

We took turns undressing each other, slowly, as I explored his adult male body, so different from my own.

I have entry after entry in my diary about my love for this man.

He told me we had to keep our romance secret because society wouldn't understand.

My love for him was all-consuming.

I spent evenings in my room fuming about the absurdity of these laws that prevented me from being with the man I loved. After all, eighteen was just an arbitrary age. I reasoned that I was far more mature than my peers. After all, I'd been helping to care for my mother through her debilitating health issues since I was seven years old.

And I was practically a surrogate wife to my step-father. I'd make his coffee in the morning and sit with him when he came home from work. I gave him massages when he was overly stressed and helped him with projects around the house.

But then I soon discovered that the man I loved was also involved with other women.

I didn't begrudge him this companionship, since we had limited opportunity to connect. We were biding our time until we could legally be together.

When I turned eighteen, I went to his apartment. I was ready for us to come out publicly as a couple and plan our wedding.

He lived in a one-bedroom apartment above a pizza parlor. It didn't even have a proper kitchen, just a half-sized fridge and toaster oven. The bathroom was down the hall, shared by other residents.

My intended husband walked me over to his bed and sat me down. I started to unbutton my blouse, but he put his hand on mine and then pulled my hand to his lips. He kissed each of my fingers, and then looked down.

"We have to end this," he said.

I don't remember what else was said. I ran from his apartment building, struggling to breathe, hysterical.

When I got home, I couldn't stop shaking. I started to think of ways to end my life.

As I was generating a plan, I remembered a card someone had given me at a health fair I'd attended a few months earlier.

It had the number of a suicide hotline.

I called the number, not because I'd decided I wanted to live, but because I needed to get information.

I had to plan my suicide so it looked like an accident. My mother had attempted suicide a number of times when I was a kid. I remember the pain it had caused my family. So I needed to figure out how to end my life in a way that looked like a hapless accident.

Whoever I spoke to on the suicide hotline that day saved my life.

It is hard for me to put into words how convinced I was that society was wrong about the age of consent. I was absolutely sure that I was capable of making a choice about being in a sexual relationship with a man twice my age.

I was so certain, that I was offended by a law that claimed I wasn't mature enough to make decisions about my sexuality.

As it turns out, I wasn't.

Now that I am an adult, I look back at myself as a love struck fourteen-year-old with some perspective. I feel compassion for myself. I was a needy, lonely, unpopular kid, who was desperate for attention and acceptance. Realizing that this man took advantage of me is painful. It is difficult to admit how wrong I was, and that my confidence in my own maturity was actually a sign of my immaturity.

One of the reasons that adolescence is a time of turmoil is that teenagers often feel like they are right, and that anybody who disagrees with them is wrong. They develop the distinctive cockiness of teenhood because they feel like they are capable of making adult decisions while they are still treated like children. Although teenagers can appear mature for their years, even the most mature teenager is still not an adult.

Deborah Yurgelun-Todd and colleagues at the McLean Hospital Brain Imaging Center in Boston, Massachusetts note that "While adults can use rational processes when facing emotional decisions, teenagers are simply not yet equipped to think through things in the same way."[156]

This is because teens' frontal lobes are still developing, meaning they tend to make decisions based on feelings, emotions, and what they want at the moment, rather than based on weighing pros and cons and long-term consequences.

As we continue to learn more about human development, we are finding out that many people don't hit developmental markers of adulthood until their mid-twenties. Eighteen is the youngest age at which someone should be considered capable of giving consent for medical interventions that have lifelong consequences.

And yet children as young as eight years old—and possibly even younger—are given puberty blockers to prevent them from developing normally. These puberty blockers retard their normal growth physically, mentally, and emotionally.

* * *

At these young ages children think in terms of black and white, they view things in extremes, and are unable to appreciate nuance. They tend to be emotionally volatile, and subject to peer pressure. They are impatient and lack the ability to plan ahead for the future. At eight years old, children still have baby teeth. They are not capable of making decisions regarding medical treatment, especially medical treatment that causes their bodies to be less healthy and functional.

Dr. Paul Hruz, a professor at Washington University School of Medicine, Lawrence Mayer, a scholar in residence at Johns Hopkins School of Medicine and Dr. Paul McHugh, of Johns Hopkins University School of Medicine, authored the article *Growing Pains: Problems with Puberty Suppression in Treating Gender Dysphoria* which raises serious concerns about the use of puberty blockers for children with gender dysphoria.

Though proponents of puberty blockers say that the effects are reversible, Hruz, Mayer and McHugh found that "there are virtually no published reports, even case studies, of adolescents withdrawing from puberty-suppressing drugs and then resuming the normal pubertal development typical for their sex."[157]

The long-term side effects for a child taking puberty blockers are unknown. No research exists because this intervention is so new.

Research on the short-term side effects of puberty blockers include loss of bone density, early onset menopause, joint pain and cognitive delays.[158, 159, 160, 161, 162, 163, 164] One study done in England showed that children taking puberty blockers had an increase in behavioral and emotional problems, self-harm, and suicidal thoughts.[165]

Dr John Gueriguian, who spent twenty years reviewing drugs for the FDA, stated in federal court papers that AbbVie, the manufacturer of Lupron, which is a commonly used puberty blocker, intentionally suppressed information about the danger associated with the use of Lupron.[166]

The FDA has an adverse-events database that lists more than 25,000 adverse events associated with Lupron, including suicidal thoughts, vision loss, and excruciating pain, as well as death.[167]

In addition to all the risks associated with puberty blockers, giving children puberty blockers encourages them to believe they are born in the wrong bodies, and greatly increases the likelihood these children will want cross-sex hormones and transgender surgeries.

Dr. Michael Biggs, a professor of sociology at Oxford found that not only did almost all the children treated with puberty blockers at the Tavistock Gender Identity Service in the United Kingdom go on to cross-sex hormones but children taking puberty blockers had an increase in self-harming behavior.

Hruz, Lawrence, and McHugh note that "Gender identity for children is elastic (that is, it can change over time) and plastic (that is, it can be shaped by forces like parental approval and social conditions)," therefore puberty blockers interfere with the natural process by which children become comfortable with themselves.

Puberty blockers don't only prevent physical maturation, they also inhibit emotional maturation. Children who have been taking puberty blockers are developmentally younger than their peers. They are consistently shown to be less emotionally mature, intellectually retarded (meaning slowed or behind their peers), and developmentally delayed.

The effects of puberty blockers are not reversible.[168, 169] A child can never recapture the time missed while peers are developing normally.[170, 171] We will not know all the negative consequence of a healthy child taking puberty blockers and cross-sex hormones until these children grow up.

Transing children is a medical experiment akin to some of the most egregious medical abuses in history, such as the frontal lobotomies and eugenics.

* * *

Children as young as eight years old are currently being given cross-sex hormones, often in conjunction with puberty blockers, which leave them not only developmentally delayed but frequently sterilized.[172]

Scarlet, who started on cross-sex hormones at thirteen and puberty blockers at fourteen, said that his reproductive organs have been so stunted that he is essentially a eunuch.

Scarlet was never told of the dangers or side effects of these interventions. Like so many other children, Scarlet was the subject of an experimental treatment, and was told it would help him with his difficult feelings. As it turns out, his difficult feelings were those of a gay boy, and not even those of a boy with gender dysphoria.[173]

And if the hormonal interventions aren't sadistic enough, surgeons go on to chop off children's healthy body parts.

Johanna Olsen-Kennedy, a prominent gender clinician and activist, insists it is no big deal to cut off a child's healthy breasts. She states that if a girl decides she isn't really transgender, or if the treatment doesn't alleviate her gender dysphoria, she can always get another pair ... of breasts.[174] Dr. Olsen-Kennedy seems not to understand the difference between breast tissue and silicone, which isn't surprising since she is also confused about the difference between male and female.

Boys as young as sixteen years old are being surgically castrated, which finishes off the work of the puberty blockers they took, which were formerly used to chemically castrate sex offenders.[175]

The doctors who currently perform mutilating transing surgeries on children justify their actions by saying that the children they operate on are mature enough to decide to undergo elective cosmetic surgery that permanently alter their bodies. If a child (or a child's parent) said he or she didn't want children, they would be hard pressed to find a surgeon who would be willing to surgically sterilize them, in fact it is even difficult for adults to find doctors who will sterilize young adults who haven't had children. In fact, even Planned Parenthood reports that "sterilization may be difficult to arrange if a person is single or childless and under 35" and "Federally funded sterilizations may not be performed on anyone under 21 or anyone incapable of legal consent."[176] And yet gender clinics are routinely sterilizing vulnerable children.

We do not fully understand the lifelong consequences of medical transitioning children because this is uncharted territory, but we do know some of the serious side effects it involves.

Common side effects from puberty blockers include:

- Redness, burning, pain, and bruising at injection site
- Hot flashes
- Increased sweating
- Night sweats
- Tiredness
- Headache
- Nausea
- Diarrhea
- Constipation
- Stomach pain
- Breast swelling or tenderness
- Acne
- Joint/muscle aches or pain
- Trouble sleeping

- Vaginal discomfort/dryness/itching/discharge
- Vaginal bleeding
- Swelling of the ankles/feet
- Increased urination at night
- Dizziness
- Weakness
- Chills
- Clammy skin
- Itching or scaling
- Testicle pain
- Impotence
- Depression
- Increased growth of facial hair
- Memory problems

Once a child starts on puberty blockers, s/he is on a direct pathway to cross-gender hormones.

Side effects of hormones given to girls to make them appear more masculine include:

- An abnormal amount of lipids in the blood
- Worsening of an underlying manic or psychotic condition
- Producing too many red blood cells (polycythemia)
- Weight gain
- Acne
- Developing male-pattern baldness
- Sleep apnea
- Elevated liver function tests
- High blood pressure
- Type 2 diabetes
- Infertility
- Extreme uterine pain

- Uterine atrophy often necessitating a hysterectomy

Hormones given to boys to make them appear more feminine also have considerable risks, including:

- A blood clot in vein or in a lung
- High triglycerides
- Gallstones
- Weight gain
- Elevated liver function tests
- Decreased libido
- Erectile dysfunction
- Infertility
- High potassium
- High blood pressure
- Type 2 diabetes
- Cardiovascular disease

In addition, medicalizing a child's healthy body causes not only physical damage, but a huge financial burden as well. Not only are the initial costs of transing high, but a child who is given these interventions faces lifelong medical costs.

Most of these children will outgrow their dysphoria if allowed to progress naturally through childhood. These children are being treated with experimental, expensive, medicalizing interventions, when the only proven cure is no intervention at all, possibly coupled with therapy.

Imagine treating any other condition that naturally resolves with interventions that cause lifelong damage. It is unthinkable, or at least it should be.

* * *

I suspect that most teenagers have something about their bodies that they would like changed. If offered cosmetic surgery, many would jump at the opportunity to "improve" their bodies, and they would likely be "happier" post-surgery, at least in the short term. But the lesson children are taught when they are told to change their bodies rather than their feelings about their bodies is that their bodies are at fault for their unhappiness. This sets them up to believe that any time one is unhappy with one's body, the only solution is to change one's body.

This is diametrically opposed to the lesson children need to be taught.

One of our lifelong challenges as human beings is resolving the expectations of how we want to look, versus what our bodies actually look like. I have never met anyone who is 100% happy with his or her body. Teenagers, especially, tend to be narcissistically preoccupied with their bodies.

Normalizing elective cosmetic surgery for teenagers reinforces the unhealthy and damaging idea that our bodies should look the way we want them to look in order for us to be able to find happiness.

Another reason that adolescence is tumultuous is that teens are constantly feeling like societal rules and expectations are making them unhappy. Adolescence is a time when children should begin to learn that happiness is a shallow, fleeting emotion. Happiness is not sustaining, it is like a sugar rush or a drug high: it feels good at the time, but does not lead to long-term emotional well-being.

One of the markers of adulthood is recognizing that life is not about being constantly happy.

Thankfully, we have laws that protect children because we know that children often focus on being happy rather than on being emotionally and physically healthy. We recognize that children need rules and guidelines to protect them from both themselves and others.

* * *

It is unfathomable that we have come to accept a situation where children are causing permanent harm to otherwise healthy bodies. It is unconscionable that transgender-rights activists are actively pushing children to medically transition, and in many states, have managed to pass legislation that prohibits children with gender dysphoria from accessing mental health care to help them resolve their gender dysphoria.

DETRANSITIONING

"One woman, very, very pointedly spoke about her eating disorder. And she said, 'and when I had my eating disorder, I was given great care and my parents gave me great care and the professionals gave me great care. You know, six months later I had gender dysphoria and within months I'd had a mastectomy. And when I left the clinic for the mastectomy, in my hand, I had a leaflet for phalloplasty.' So it was like, the clinics were almost selling her further surgeries."

—Stella O'Malley
A speaker at the world's first detransition conference[177]

The same doctors who insist that children with gender dysphoria will kill themselves if they don't medically transition, dismiss the intense feelings of discomfort detransitioners have due to changes brought on by transing.

Girls and women develop a deep voice, an enlarged Adam's apple, facial and body hair, a receding hairline, and an enlarged clitoris from masculinizing hormones. Boys develop breasts. Those who have had surgeries are missing body parts they can never replace.

Instead of admitting that distress over these bodily changes is as concerning as the original distress that resulted in these kids being pushed to transition, doctors, therapists, trans-rights activists, and people in the culture have been brainwashed to follow along and tell detransitioners to "buck up."

In testimony before the Utah legislature, Dr. Nicole Mihalopoulos said, "If for some reason, five years later, your child says, 'You know what dad? Hm. I dunno if that was exactly the right thing for me,' in referring to taking puberty blockers and/or hormones, and/or having surgery, they can stop their medicine. There are going to be some changes that are considered semi-permanent of those, a thickening of the vocal-chords, which causes voice deepening."

Mihalopoulos notes that there are many people who don't like their voices and have an option of engaging in voice training to change their voice.

She goes on to say that an increase in body hair is another permanent change but minimizes any distress a detransitioner might feel about her five o'clock shadow or hairy chest by saying, "Well, oh my gosh. There are lots of cis-gender women who have lots of body hair and facial hair. I'm Greek. I, we spend a lot of money on hair removal."[178]

This is a typical response detransitioners get when they express discomfort over the changes medical transing has done to them.

So the question is, why is it that when someone is uncomfortable with his or her natural voice, body hair and/or other secondary sex characteristics, that person is rushed to transition, but if he or she detransitions, the message is to deal with the discomfort?

If a person suffers with discomfort for any other reason besides gender dysphoria, that person is generally told that feelings of discomfort are a normal and natural part of life. But today everyone is coerced into believing that if children and teens are not able to change their body the way they want, these children will likely kill themselves. That same discomfort is dismissed and even mocked when expressed by a detransitioner.

To add insult to injury, these detransitioners were told by health care professionals that transing would "cure" their feelings of discomfort, and that transing was the only treatment path. They were told they would likely become suicidal and might even kill themselves if they didn't transition. But then when they realized that transing didn't cure them, the same doctors dismiss their feelings of distress and have nothing else to offer them.

Elie Vandenbussche examined the needs of detransitioners. In her study *Detransition-Related Needs and Support*, Vandenbussche found that nearly 80% or those who responded to her study reported they were not properly informed about the health implications of the transing interventions their health care provider was recommending.[179]

To make the process of detransitioning even more difficult, those who detransition have very little support. Often they are ostracized by the very community that welcomed and celebrated them as transgender.

Josh Drewes described his experience. "The thing is with the culture simply coming out, it's celebrated," but he says when he detransitioned the same people who celebrated his trans identity "abandoned me."[180]

When I speak publicly about my experience as a former "trans" kid, the hostility expressed by those who claim to be tolerant and loving is shocking. They insist that my gender dysphoria must not have been very bad. They claim that I have internalized transphobia. And they will insist that I was never really trans.

For people who demand to define themselves and who demand that everyone else capitulate to their demands, these hypocrites have no problem dismissing anyone else's experience if the experience does not support their narrative.

Willow was transed as a child. After detransitioning, she was told, "You weren't ever really trans, you know, fake trans versus a real one. You weren't really a real trans person," despite her deep voice, five o-clock shadow, and enlarged Adam's apple, all the result of having taken testosterone.

Willow warns that many detransitioners are silent due to being bullied and intimidated by trans-rights activists. She says that they "are scared to come out as detransitioners publicly."[181]

The irony is that the claim, "You were never really trans," is actually a compelling argument against transing kids at all. If a child who was so determinedly certain of having a trans identity can later change his or her mind—as many do—then no child should ever be transed.

Willow and I are just two of many examples proving that although children can suffer from crippling gender dysphoria, that doesn't mean we were born in the wrong body, we were inherently flawed, and/or that we must transition or we will die by suicide.

The number of detransitioners is on the rise, because children and young adults are being denied appropriate mental health services. Instead they are told that transing will cure their distress, and they are being lied to about the consequences of medical transition.

Sydney Wright didn't know she had any other option but medical transition. She says, "It's not known how many detransitioners like me exist, but there are lots of us. All have similar stories of medical abuse, medical mutilation, and no real treatment options other than medical transition."[182]

As Rachel Foster says, "Pushing a person like myself in that direction and encouraging that person to take medical steps, I think was a very dangerous thing. I was not told about much of the long-term effects from my therapist."

Rachel was never told of the debilitating side effects brought on by cross-sex hormones. She found out the hard way. "After almost five years on testosterone, I started to experience liver and kidney failure. However, I was not prepared or told even that kidney and liver damage could be related to cross sex hormones."[183]

Neither was Kevin warned about the consequences of taking cross-sex hormones. "When I was trans, nothing worked down there. Well, it was painful. And like it shrank a lot, and everything just—nothing worked properly. And it was painful. Sex hurt. It was not pleasureful for me, it hurt. I didn't like it."

Kevin detransitioned after realizing that his quality of life had not improved by transing.[184]

YouTuber Rival Maverick reflects on how easy it was to get testosterone and how little she really understood what was happening. "I wasn't given any information. I mean, they're pretty much just like, 'Here's your prescription, you know, you can be on your way.'"[185]

Leoaica Motanelul shared how distressing her process of detransitioning was. After doing everything she could conceive of, from hormones, to mastectomy, to a hysterectomy, she finally realized that transing didn't help. This was a troubling realization: "And so I was just like, wow, okay, this is it. This is the end of the road. That was the last surgery I was going to get. So what do I do if I'm not getting another surgery? There's nothing to look forward to."

Once she realized that transing wasn't the answer to her difficult feelings, she said, "the depression hit me really hard. And I was like, I'm still not happy. I'm still not happy after all of this."

And to top it all off, she discovered that the surgery she underwent might have irreversible consequences. "I started doing research and I found some really terrifying statistics that like women had 200 percent more risk of developing dementia and heart attacks and stroke when they had had these hysterectomies that removed not only the uterus, but their ovaries as well. And I got terrified by that."[186]

Billy Burleigh was also left with inconceivable damage. Like so many detransitioners, he is permanently medicalized. Though he has a positive outlook for someone who has been through so much he acknowledges, "In order for me to be healthy, just stay healthy, I need testosterone and I have to inject it every week. So I have to turn around and give myself a shot in the rear end every week."[187]

Children who are put on puberty blockers and then cross-sex hormones, who are put on cross-sex hormones at a young age, and who undergo surgery to remove sex organs generally become unable to produce the hormones their bodies need to stay healthy and functional. For girls it is like they went through menopause. Boys become much like eunuchs. These kids must either remain transed and take cross-sex hormones for the rest of their lives, or detransition and take synthetic hormones for the rest of their lives.

Imagine taking children who are physically healthy and damaging them to the point where they have to take artificial hormones for the rest of their lives. This is not only unethical, it is expensive, putting these children at risk of being destitute as a result of being transed as children. Forcing children into making this choice benefits only one group: the pharmaceutical companies.

It is difficult to believe that children and young adults are pushed on a path of permanent medical transitioning rather than encouraged to address the underlying causes of their dysphoria.

James Caspian wanted to study the experience of detransitioners after he talked to Dr. Miro Djordjevic, a surgeon who performs transing surgeries. Dr. Djordjevic mentioned that he had seen an unprecedented number of people who had transed come back to him to see if he could reverse the surgeries.

Caspian wanted to study this phenomenon, but was told by his department that he wouldn't be allowed because it "might attract criticism on social media, and criticism of the research would be criticism of the university. And furthermore, it is better not to offend people."[188]

A belief system has become more important than science.

The travesty is that those who detransition still have to process the original underlying issues that led to their gender dysphoria; but they must also process their grief over the damage transing did to their bodies, over the realization that they were betrayed by the very people who were supposed to help them, as well as deal with the abandonment they experienced from the community that originally affirmed them.

It is heartbreaking to hear stories of those who believed with all their heart that transitioning via medical interventions would cure them, but then they discovered that not only did the interventions not cure them, they were also left with other significant problems, such as debilitating side effects from the drugs and surgical scars. In many cases, detransitioners have been medicalized for life, suffering surgical complications and the need for hormones to replace those that their body would have naturally created prior to being transed.

Billy captures this horrifying predicament. After taking hormones, having his penis cut off and inverted, having his face feminized, his voice box stitched, and his Adam's apple shaved, he recognized that nothing had improved. "I knew all of the books, all of the medical research that I read, all the journal articles and everything else that I read that said I needed to change my body to match my mind. My mind wasn't changing. My body had changed, but I had other problems... I had other problems it seemed like that this wasn't addressing, this wasn't solving."[189] He goes on to say, "I had more problems then, than I had at the beginning of the transition journey."

These problems are two-fold for many detransitioners.

Transing prevented them from addressing the underlying issues that caused the gender dysphoria in the first place. All that time wasted on transition could have been spent getting help for those underlying issues.

In addition, their bodies are damaged.

Billy realized his gender dysphoria was caused by a combination of his learning disability, his physical build, and a sexual assault. As a result of transing, he is no longer able to experience an orgasm. He lost his ability to consummate his marriage, to enjoy a healthy sex life, to father a child.

Ashira is faced with a similar reality. She thought that transing would cure her difficulties, but later realized that autism was causing her distress. She says, "I had a top surgery, and unfortunately I had a hysterectomy and oophorectomy, so, uh, I can't have babies." This loss causes her deep sadness now that she has detransitioned.[190]

Leoaica who had her breasts and uterus removed says, "I had this intense grief. I was so angry at myself for having made this decision and I was angry at the doctors for having let me. They removed perfectly healthy organs. I got everything out. I got my cervix, my uterus, my fallopian tubes, my ovaries, I got everything removed. There's nothing in there—perfectly healthy organs that I just decided to get rid of."

She goes on to say "I made a really dangerous choice that I have to live with. I have to live with this for the rest of my life and it terrifies me. So honestly, I just try not to think about it."[191]

But Leoaica and other detransitioners need to remember that they didn't make a choice; they were put on a path by those pushing mystical beliefs about gender onto vulnerable children. They were told that there was no way to manage or resolve their difficult feelings without transing.

They were not given any other treatment options.

Now that they have realized that transing wasn't a cure, they are left to pick up the pieces—often alone, as they have been rejected by their community—while being told by doctors like Dr. Nicole Mihalopoulos that the irreversible damage done to them is no big deal.[192]

DISMISSING & DISPARAGING
DETRANSITIONERS

"Thoroughly talk through your mental health and any hang-ups you have with a therapist, and make sure that you are as certain as possible that you are transitioning because it is what you need rather than as a way to avoid dealing with something else. No matter how well you think you know yourself, brains are tricky jerks. I know several detransitioners who feel they would have been a lot better off if they had put a little more effort into looking at the things bothering them rather than skipping straight to DIY [do it yourself] hormones."

—Disposabletag2*

Transgender-rights activists dismiss and disparage people like me, who had gender dysphoria and learned how to manage or resolve it without transitioning, as well as those who transitioned and then detransitioned.

They dismiss and disparage us because we are living evidence that gender dysphoria can be managed and resolved in ways other than transitioning.

We are living testimony that transitioning children is not an appropriate treatment for childhood gender dysphoria.

We are proof that gender dysphoric children do not need to be and should not be transitioned.

Our ongoing lives demonstrate that gender dysphoric children don't inevitably kill themselves if they do not transition.

* * *

ShatterHawk is careful about who she tells her story to because of the response she's endured from the transgender community. "I can completely relate to realizing that my dysphoria had actual causes that could be identified and healed. Unfortunately, I can't talk about this with my trans friends, since it is often interpreted as a justification for 'conversion therapy.' I also was able to get a diagnosis at an early age, but my parent's gently encouraged me to wait. I'm glad that I did, since a medical transition would have been disastrous for my mental and physical health. It scares me that it is so strongly pushed forward as THE ONLY CURE for dysphoric young women."

Rather than hear stories like these and advocate for more research and treatment options for children with gender dysphoria, transgender-rights activists try to pretend that those like me and ShatterHawk don't exist.

But we do. And our stories need to be heard.

I have been told by transgender-rights activists that it isn't possible to resolve or manage gender dysphoria. They say that I am not actually a woman who struggled with gender dysphoria, but I am, in fact, a gay man trapped in a woman's body who is transphobic because I have not transitioned.

This is an interesting spin, which suggests that it is better to be less functional and to attempt to transition sexes, than to be more functional and admit that gender dysphoria is treatable.

Others who speak publicly about their detransition are also treated with contempt.

Stormy Z says that a lot of times, detransitioners don't talk about it "because the LGBTQ+ community treats detransitioners appallingly. They're told to shut up, to stop discouraging transitioners, they're told they were 'never really trans in the first place,' or that their detransition only gives Christian fundamentalists hate fuel. Detransitioners often report losing all of their LGBTQ+ friends and even receive hate or death threats. So beautiful, considering it comes from the same community that preaches that all love is love."

Ryptoll talks about her detransitioning, "The majority of the trans community would shun me now. They often view detransitioners as a threat, I've noticed, and try to silence us."

Another detransitioner said, "I recently lost my entire friend group. So I go to college but I lost all of my friends."

Leo says, "I was on T (testosterone) for a year before realizing it wasn't for me." Leo goes on to explain how the transgender community tries to silence anyone who has detransitioned, saying there is "so much hate for it."

The Atlantic featured the story of Carey Callahan. "After years of harassment and discomfort in her female body, she had made the decision to transition to being male. In the short term, she was happy. But she soon discovered that life as a transgender man was not what she had expected. Her discomfort persisted, as did the harassment." Carey says that "detransitioning has resulted in the most harassment" she has ever faced.[193]

Cass, a thirty-one-year-old detransitioned lesbian says, "There are a significant number of trans people and trans allies who find what I and other detransitioned people have to say threatening or dangerous, and they would rather we not say. Trans people sometimes treat detransitioned people more as symbols of what they fear than as real people."

Bondiee captures the current narrative of transgender-rights activists: "Today, we are told that those with gender dysphoria—whether they are four-year-old children or Olympic athletes—are better off living as the opposite sex."

She also describes the consequences of unquestioningly acceptance of this treatment approach:

> Putting blind trust in those who use bullying tactics to discourage debate or scientific challenge has traumatic and sometimes deadly consequences for the innocent victims. Consider the harm that occurs today as a result of this propaganda: Unbiased medical information and treatment is simply not available to those considering sex change. Only one course of treatment is provided: hormone treatment and sex reassignment surgery. Hurting people who regret transitioning are bullied into silence. Researchers can be run out of their profession if their results challenge the transgender-rights activists' narrative. The freedom to pursue scientific evidence is in jeopardy.

Bondiee goes on to question the idea that anyone with gender dysphoria should transition:

> Let's stop enabling the delusion that transition is the only answer. Let's allow scientific research to flourish, no matter what the results show. Let's look at the evidence and facts and encourage treatment options that address dangerous psychiatric conditions first. In that way, we can ensure the best outcomes for those who have gender dysphoria. People with a diagnosis of gender dysphoria are encouraged to undergo sex transition as treatment. But according to studies, over half of this population is likely to have one or more coexisting psychiatric disorders, such as depression, phobias, and adjustment disorders, which influence the outcomes. The coexisting psychiatric disorders should be treated first before undergoing irreversible, life-changing sex change surgeries. Yet any report of psychiatric issues among transgenders is seen as too negative to the social justice narrative. Individuals with gender dysphoria are discouraged from seeking treatment for their depression, phobias, and adjustment disorders. Instead, it is assumed that their psychiatric difficulties are due to their "not being true to themselves," and they are fast-tracked to transition. To my knowledge, transgender advocates have never made a point to warn the transgender community to look for other treatable disorders or to lobby the medical community for better diagnosis and care for coexisting disorders, which are present in over half the group.

Those of us who try to tell our stories about overcoming or managing gender dysphoria are bullied. Our experiences are disregarded. We are told that we "converted," that we have internalized transphobia, and that we can't understand being transgender because obviously we really weren't really transgender. We are also told that our gender dysphoria must have been minor.

Though all of these responses are meant to bolster transgender-rights activists' claim that children with gender dysphoria should transition, each of these responses actually undermines their claim.

Trans-rights activists claim that a child knows if he or she is transgender, that it is immutable and unchanging. So every time someone speaks out saying, "Wait a minute, I was sure I was trans and I was wrong," it calls attention to a foundational flaw in the transgender ideology and undermines the narrative supporting medical interventions for transing children.

APPENDIX A:
GROOMING & RECRUITMENT AT SCHOOL

Gender ideology has become part of the atmosphere in public schools. The website genderspectrum.org[194] had in its "Toolkit" a description of the four "Entry Points" by which activists could get gender ideology into schools:

1. **Internal Entry Point:** Changing how people think about gender
2. **Interpersonal Entry Point:** Changing how people talk to each other about gender
3. **Instructional Entry Point:** Getting gender ideology into every single classroom
4. **Institutional Entry Point:** Putting into place policies that solidify gender ideology as a permanent fixture in schools

(Gender Spectrum has since removed this from their site, but screenshots are available at https://arlingtonparentcoa.wixsite.com/arlingtonparentcoa/what-schools-are-doing.)[195]

Trans-rights activists have successfully achieved entree via the first three entry points, and are now succeeding at the fourth with laws like H.R. 5 (the so-called "Equality Act", which replaces "sex" with "gender identity," effectively erasing the biological categories of male and female) and GLSEN's Model School District Policy,[196] which is being funneled into every school in the nation.

On a day-to-day level, children pre-K through 12 are exposed to and brainwashed into gender ideology via:

- books[197]
- curriculum designed to promote it in every subject[198]

- Peer-Led Sex Ed[199]
- posters on the walls and classroom doors[200]
- teachers inserting gender ideology into their classes[201]
- counselors leading children to question their gender identity[202]
- Gay-Straight Alliance / Gender Sexuality Alliance clubs[203]
- plays about "gender diverse" characters[204]
- assemblies & guest speakers promoting LGB & TQ issues[205]
- special holidays like "National Coming Out Day" and "Transgender Day of Remembrance" nearly every month of the school year[206]
- promotion of LGB & TQ events and interests[207]
- policies that enforce acceptance of transgender ideology[208]

Via the vehicle of Critical Race Theory (CRT) it is impressed upon children that being white, "cis" (having one's internal sense of identity match his/her biology), and heterosexual is the very worst thing one can be. White, cis, het males are the worst of oppressors, according to CRT, and the most virtuous people are those who are most oppressed; therefore it behooves children to adopt victim status.

Interestingly, adopting a transgender identity is a very easy way to become "marginalized" for kids whose skin color and background do not otherwise lend themselves to appearing oppressed. Furthermore, once a child says that s/he is transgender, that child is untouchable: no one may question or criticize anything the child says, wants, or does. A transgender student can have a teacher fired.[209] That's a heady amount of power for a child.

If a child is in a public school today, that child is being indoctrinated into sexuality and gender ideologies that are intended to make the child fodder for the gender industry's medicalization machine. This is a billion-dollar business.[210]

* * *

How has transgender ideology taken over the schools, the healthcare industry, and the culture so quickly and comprehensively? Besides sneaking in on the coattails of the LGB and the civil rights movements, TQ activism has also carried out one incredibly diabolical scheme: vilifying good parents as child abusers.

In her book *Desist, Detrans, & Detox: Getting Your Child Out of the Gender Cult,*[211] Maria Keffler outlines myriad harms that the gender industry perpetrates on children and families. One of the most malevolent is the predatory child-grooming tactics it copies straight from the pedophile playbook:

One of the most powerful predictors of academic success is parental involvement,[212] and the most significant force for stability in a society is the intact nuclear family.[213] No adults are more influential in a child's life than his or her parents. No other relationship, save potentially with a spouse, will have as long a history, as deep a present, and as far-reaching a future in that child's life. The parent-child relationship has been respected and honored throughout human history and across cultures.

Until now.

When something or someone seeks to sever or come between the relationship between a parent and child, except in cases of extreme parental neglect or abuse, that separation is almost always enacted for nefarious reasons, often resulting in victimization of the child.[214] Isolating a child from parents or guardians is one of the calculated steps that pedophiles and predators take in order to groom a child for sexual abuse.[215]

One such tactic is revealed in the below excerpt from the *New Yorker.* Malcolm Gladwell relates psychologist Carla van Dam's story about her work with former teacher and convicted pedophile Jeffrey Clay.

Clay … first put himself in a place with easy access to children—an elementary school. Then he worked his way through his class. He began by simply asking boys if they wanted to stay after school. "Those who could not do so without parental permission were screened out," van Dam writes. Children with vigilant parents are too risky.[216]

Think about that: "Children with vigilant parents are too risky." What's risky? The risk to the child abuser is that he *gets caught abusing the child.*

We've already seen that in-school gender activists are actively pursuing vulnerable kids in order to lure them into the gender cult.[217] Gender & Sexuality Allies club leaders admit they poach kids from the counseling office.[218] GLSEN,[219] Human Rights Campaign's Welcoming Schools program,[220] the American School Counselor Association,[221] and increasing numbers of school districts have codified their determination to keep sex and gender information about children from the children's own parents.[222]

We've seen counselors and therapists break some of the most basic ethics espoused by their licensing boards. From the Social Workers Code of Ethics:

Social workers seek to strengthen relationships among people in a purposeful effort to promote, restore, maintain, and enhance the well-being of individuals, *families,* social groups, organizations, and communities," and "Social workers should not take unfair advantage of any professional relationship to exploit others *to further their personal, religious, political, or business interests.*[223]

Social media gender influencers and self-styled "glitter-moms" tell kids to ditch their own families and come hook up with them.[224]

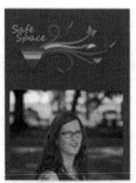

I want you to know that it's okay to walk away from unsupportive or disrespectful or even abusive parents. And I want to give you hope that you can find what we call your glitter family. Your queer family. **We are out there.**

And the relationships we make in our glitter families are just as real, just as meaningful as our blood families.

(Text above is verbatim, but was re-created for visual clarity.)

We've seen parents lose custody of their own biological children because they won't provide wrong-sex hormones.[225] We've seen a father go to prison[226] for not protecting the identity of a doctor who coaches kids to threaten suicide in order to get puberty blockers, wrong-sex hormones, and surgery.[227] We've seen a boarding school principal arrange for an underage boy to undergo a sex change operation, behind his mother's back.[228]

What do all of these events, the likes of which are beginning to snowball into an avalanche of catastrophe for children and families, have in common? Loving and concerned parents were circumvented and/or undermined so the child could be victimized by the profit-driven gender industry.

Make no mistake, gender medicine and politics is exactly as loving, kind, and supportive as a pedophile molesting a helpless child in the restroom.

In fact, child molesters and the gender industry do and say exactly the same things. Compare school districts' transgender-student policies with child predator tactics:

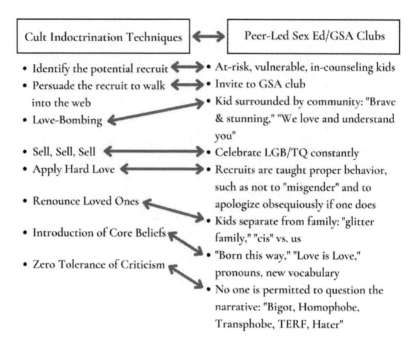

Cult Indoctrination Techniques	Peer-Led Sex Ed/GSA Clubs
• Identify the potential recruit	• At-risk, vulnerable, in-counseling kids
• Persuade the recruit to walk into the web	• Invite to GSA club
• Love-Bombing	• Kid surrounded by community: "Brave & stunning," "We love and understand you"
• Sell, Sell, Sell	• Celebrate LGB/TQ constantly
• Apply Hard Love	• Recruits are taught proper behavior, such as not to "misgender" and to apologize obsequiously if one does
• Renounce Loved Ones	• Kids separate from family: "glitter family," "cis" vs. us
• Introduction of Core Beliefs	• "Born this way," "Love is Love," pronouns, new vocabulary
• Zero Tolerance of Criticism	• No one is permitted to question the narrative: "Bigot, Homophobe, Transphobe, TERF, Hater"

There's no neutral middle-ground when it comes to the gender industry. One either recognizes the harms and fights for parents' authority and children's protections, or one is complicit in the industry's predatory profiteering and active destruction of children and their families.

CONCLUSION

"In 15, 20 years, the science of all this is going to be so clear and so laid out and it will be just like the lobotomy movement. And everyone will be looking back saying, 'Oh, how is this possible? How could this, you know, how savage these people were kind of thing,' but until then there are lives to be rescued and it's not, you know, they're not being rescued by transition affirming therapy."

—Dr. Andre Van Mol[229]

I recently heard about another young woman who is transing. She wants a more pronounced Adam's apple, so she consulted with a surgeon about the possibility of having a chunk of her rib removed and transferred to her neck. The surgeon is considering it.

Researchers are already investigating the possibility of transplanting a uterus into a man to make him feel more like a woman, and perhaps even gestate a baby.

What about a fake prostate?

All this time, money, and effort is going into damaging children while we have children who are lacking basic health care, food, and housing.

We are willing to make a healthy child unhealthy while sick children can't get basic care, hungry children are unable to find food, and cold children don't have anywhere to live.

"Transgender medicine" is a scandal and a disgrace.

* * *

To suggest that children who struggle with gender dysphoria be affirmed by therapists is to agree that transitioning is a healthier and more desirable outcome. Nothing could be further from the truth.

Children who transition are more likely to have long-term mental and physical health challenges as a result of transitioning.

Transing a child indicates that one subscribes to a belief that there is such a thing as an innate gender—a gender spirit—that can inhabit the wrong body. It affirms the idea that there is an appropriate way for children to express gender identity, and that a child who does not adhere to traditional gender norms is inherently flawed, or in other words, transgender.

* * *

Historically schools have taught kids how to handle peer pressure. It can be hard to be a kid who wants to feel a part of a group to say "no" to something the group demands. And this, I think, is at the heart of the sudden jump in children who are being transed.

For a kid who doesn't fit in, transgender-rights activists provide support groups, clubs, and advocates; all the kid has to do is say s/he is genderfluid, gender non-conforming, gender non-binary, transgender, or gender confused. That kid who didn't fit in now has friends, allies, and acceptance. The less the kid conforms to social norms and is victimized by others, the more support he or she will get from transgender-rights activists.

As kids hit milestones in their transition, others in the group celebrate and encourage them towards the next step. First a kid decides to change her name, then her gender pronouns, then officially transition both at home and at school. Next she starts puberty blockers, then cross-sex hormones, and finally invasive surgery.

All along the way, members of the community are cheering her on.

The community might even hold fundraisers for her so she can afford what can only be described as elective cosmetic medical interventions.

These kids are encouraged to focus so much on themselves, and their right to express themselves, that they become increasingly fixated on how they look.

Though teens and young adults generally are concerned about their appearance, it is hard to conceive of any other situation in which a child would be encouraged to medically alter his or her body with dangerous experimental interventions, just to force that body to look different.

When I see threads from teens and young adults announcing that they either are about to, or just completed transition surgery, the comment threads are a love fest.

"Congratulations!"

"You are so brave, and you are loved."

"You look amazing!" and on and on.

After transitioning, or starting puberty blockers, or hormones, or surgery, these young people are also enticed by their community to document their victimhood. Instances where someone deadnamed them (or used the name they were given at birth), misgendered them (mistook them for a gender other than the one they identify as), or failed to use their preferred pronouns are considered assault.

They are comforted by their group, told how brave they are, and encouraged to feel like they have been traumatized. They are also encouraged to be enraged at the way they are treated.

We have adults grooming kids to question their identities, to become hyper-focused on how their bodies look, to use unapproved medical interventions, to believe that their bodies are not okay, and to consider themselves victims.

These activists exclude and vilify anyone who does not accept their rhetoric. They provide a support system for kids and young adults who follow their approved path, but reject anyone who deviates. And they deny that another path that doesn't involve risky drugs and surgery even exists.

None of the transgender-rights activists' work promotes health or well-being.

* * *

Transgender-rights activists have done an impressive job of silencing those of us who have a personal understanding of gender dysphoria. But despite being bullied and threatened, we are sharing our stories now, because we are horrified that children with gender dysphoria are being denied mental health services, that children with gender dysphoria are being encouraged to believe that they are inherently flawed and the only way they can survive is to transition, that children with gender dysphoria are being given drugs that have not been approved for healthy children's bodies, and that children's bodies are being maimed by surgeons.

Children struggling with gender dysphoria need us. They need us to fight for their right to bodily integrity. They need us to demand that they get appropriate health services. They need us to shout from the roof-tops over and over and over again: "No child is born in the wrong body."

RESOURCES

Arlington Parent Coalition
https://www.arlingtonparentcoa.wixsite.com/arlingtonparentcoa

11th Hour Blog: https://www.the11thhourblog.com/

Commonsense Care
https://www.youtube.com/playlist?list=PLPM5Sjop1VBspuUwXd4tg
kg1UOPVDKzZi

Erin Brewer's YouTube Channel:
https://www.youtube.com/c/ErinBrewer/videos

Gender Dysphoria Support Network
https://genderdysphoriasupportnetwork.com/

Inspired Teen Therapy (Sasha Ayad, M. Ed., LPC)
https://inspiredteentherapy.com/

Irreversible Damage: The Transgender Craze Seducing Our Daughters
Abigail Shrier

Parent Resource Guide (Minnesota Family Council)
https://www.mfc.org/request-the-parent-resource-guide

Parents of ROGD Kids (Support Group Network)
https://www.parentsofrogdkids.com/

Partners for Ethical Care
https://www.partnersforethicalcare.com

Rethink Identity Medicine Ethics, Inc.
https://www.rethinkime.org/

Society for Evidence-Based Gender Medicine
https://www.segm.org/

Transgender Trend
(Questioning the Trans Narrative)
https://www.transgendertrend.com/

Truth Is The New Hate Speech
https://www.youtube.com/c/ErinBrewer/videos

Understanding Transgender Issues (Family Watch International)
https://www.familywatch.org/transgenderissues/

When Harry Became Sally: Responding to the Transgender Moment
Ryan T. Anderson

ABOUT THE AUTHORS

Erin Brewer grew up in Salt Lake City where she had inspiring high-school teachers who took the time to teach her more than academics.

She went on to earn a B.S. from Hampshire College. After getting her Master's and PhD from Utah State University, she was a stay-at-home mom and homeschool teacher for about ten years.

During this time she also volunteered at a number of local agencies and ran her own produce business.

She is co-founder of the Compassion Coalition, an international group for those fighting to ban invasive, harmful, unproven medical interventions for gender confused children; as well as Partners for Ethical Care and Advocates Protecting Children organizations that raises awareness and supports efforts to stop the unethical treatment of children by schools, hospitals, and mental and medical healthcare providers under the duplicitous banner of gender identity affirmation.

Her blog can be found at:

http://www.chooseyourowndiagnosis.com/

Maria Keffler is a co-founder of Partners for Ethical Care and Advocates Protecting Children, organizations seeking to halt the unethical medicalization of children for profit. Ms. Keffler is also a co-founder of the Arlington Parent Coalition, a watchdog group in Arlington, VA, which works to safeguard parents' rights and children's safety in public education. An author, speaker, and teacher with a background in educational psychology, Ms. Keffler lives in Arlington, Virginia (USA), with her husband and three teenagers.

GLOSSARY

The following terms are defined as the author understands their use, but not necessarily as LGB & TQ organizations would claim they are defined. Definitions are pulled from LGB & TQ materials, dictionaries, and/or the personal experience of the author.

Ally: a person who supports all LGB & TQ issues and ideologies; this is becoming more and more subjective, as many transgender-rights activists argue that homosexuals are transphobic if they refuse to date transgender-identified people who claim to be their preferred sex partners.

Androgynous: of indeterminate sex; having characteristics of both maleness and femaleness.

Antagonists: as used in this book, people who are leading your child deeper into the gender cult.

Asexual: lacking any sexual attractions to others.

Biological Sex: the sex that one was born, male or female, as evidenced by chromosomes, external anatomy (genitals, breasts), and internal anatomy (sex glands and organs).

Biphobia: prejudice against bisexual people. In current vernacular this term is applied to anyone who disagrees with anything that a bisexual person says, wants, or believes.

Bisexual: experiencing sexual attraction to both males and females.

Cis-: a prefix indicating that one's behavior or preferences align with typical or biological expectations (cisgender, cis-sexual, cis-man, etc.); this is a pejorative and nonsensical term, since no one feels completely comfortable with his or her body at all times.

Cisgender: a person whose gender identity aligns with his or her birth sex. Near antonym to **Queer**.

Closeted: an LGB/TQ person who hides his or her sexuality and/or gender identity from most other people. Antonym of **Living Openly**.

Coming Out: used as a verb or a noun, "coming out" means announcing one's sexuality or gender identity publicly.

Deadname: the name parents gave to a child when s/he was born, which is rejected in favor of a self-chosen transgender name.

Desister: a person who believed him- or herself to be transgender, but has since accepted his or her birth sex as reality.

Detransitioner: a person who presented as other than his or her birth sex, transitioning socially and/or medically, but has since accepted his or her birth sex as reality, and presents as such.

Fantasy Defense: a sexual predator's claim that he did not intend to carry out sexual activities, but was merely indulging in harmless fantasy, and/or that the victim misconstrued fantasy for reality: "It never actually happened."

FTM: Female to male transgender. Opposite of **MTF**.

Gay: homosexual, or attracted to members of one's own sex. Usually applied to males, but not exclusively.

Gender Clinic: a center that engages in experimental medical interventions where nearly every client is deemed appropriate for sex transition and assisted in attempted social and medical transition to a different sex.

Gender Dysphoria: a diagnostic term describing when one's sense of his/her gender identity does not always and/or fully match his/her biological sex.

Gender-Expansive: a term related to the ideology that gender is on a spectrum, and that one can be located anywhere on that spectrum.

Gender Expression: one's external presentation of one's gender identity; dressing and behaving like a particular sex or combination of the sexes, based upon stereotypes.

Gender-Fluid: not ascribing to one fixed gender; one whose sense of gender identity changes all the time.

Gender Identity: a nonsensical term referring to one's self-perception as male, female, or something in between; based entirely on stereotypes.

Gender-Nonconforming: not aligning with stereotypes of one's biological sex.

Genderqueer: someone who embraces gender fluidity, who doesn't present according to biological sex stereotypes. Near synonym to **Non-Binary**.

Gender Transition: attempting to change sexes (or gender expression) or to impersonate another sex (or gender expression) via social transition (dressing according to stereotypes of a different sex) or medical transition (taking puberty blockers and/or cross-sex hormones, and/or having surgeries). Gender Transition is an attempt to make the body align with the mind.

Glitter Families: older transgender-identified people who groom children to reject their families of origin and consider the transgender-identified adults their new families.

GLSEN: Gay, Lesbian, & Straight Education Network; organization creating and disseminating homosexuality and transgenderism propaganda, policy, and curricula.

Grooming: specific strategies used by child predators to gain access to children for their sexual exploitation.

Homophobia: fear or hatred of people who are same-sex attracted.

Homosexual: attracted to people of the same sex as oneself. Synonym to **Gay** and **Same-Sex Attracted**.

HRC: The Human Rights Campaign Foundation; the funding and lobby organization for the homosexual and transgender communities.

Intersex: in popular, current usage, a person who was born with mixed anatomical features of maleness and femaleness. In one recent study, the sex of a newborn was not clear from inspection of genitalia in about 1 in 1000 births. These babies have *disorders of sexual development*. Chromosomes and internal organs can be evaluated to clarify a child's sex. Some disorders of sexual development might not be discovered until puberty or after.

Lesbian: a woman who is sexually attracted to other women.

LGBTQ: An acronym for Lesbian, Gay, Bisexual, Transgender, and Queer.

LGB & TQ: An acronym for Lesbian, Gay, & Bisexual, Transgender, and Queer which delineates the very different populations of LGB people and TQ people.

Living Openly: describes those who do not hide their sexuality and/or gender identities. Antonym of **Closeted**.

Misgendering: calling someone by a pronoun they do not prefer (i.e., the biologically and grammatically correct pronoun or title).

MTF: Male to female transgender. Opposite of **FTM**.

Non-Binary: Someone who does not view himself or herself as aligning with either maleness or femaleness. Near synonym to **Genderqueer**.

Outing: (verb) revealing another person's sexuality and/or gender identity without permission to do so.

Pansexual: sexually attracted to anyone at any time; willing to be sexual partners with anyone.

Peak: (verb) recognizing that gender ideology is unsound; becoming gender-critical.

Pedophile: an adult who is sexually attracted to prepubescent children; pedophilia is still considered a mental disorder.

Polyamory: multiple (more than two) sexual partners in relationship with each other at one time.

Presentation (or Present [v]): how one shows him or herself to the world; the clothing, hairstyle, and mannerism choices that reflect one's gender (sex) status, based on cultural stereotypes.

Pronouns (also **Preferred Pronouns**): the grammatical reference used in place of a proper noun; transgender persons demand to be referred to by different pronouns that would be linguistically accurate (*e.g.*, a man tells you that his pronouns are "she/her").

Protagonists: as used in this book, people who are working with you to help pull your child out of the gender cult.

Queer: an umbrella term to express any sexual and/or gender orientation/presentation other than being a **Cisgender** heterosexual. Near antonym to **Cisgender**.

Questioning: describes someone who is exploring his or her sexuality and/or gender.

Safe Person/Space: indicates a person, place, or group that will affirm the child in transition and medicalization, and is willing to deceive/undermine parents toward that goal.

Same-Sex Attracted: attracted to people of the same sex as oneself. Synonym to **Homosexual**. Near synonym to **Gay** (males) and **Lesbian** (females).

Sex Assigned at Birth: one's biological sex. This term has been created to propagate the false idea that there is no such thing as biological sex, only the gender that someone (a doctor or parent) "assigned" to a child based on the child's genitalia.

Sexual Orientation: the nature of one's sexual and/or romantic attractions. LGB/TQ organizations often claim that sexual orientation is inherent and immutable, but this assertion is belied by the number of people who "come out" as homosexual in middle age or beyond, and those who became or returned to being heterosexual after counseling and/or therapy.

Stereotype: a widely-held idea or image of a person, which is fixed and oversimplified: e.g., "all girls like pink", "all boys like sports", "women can't do math", etc.

Supportive: willing to capitulate to all demands of the transgender-identified person.

TERF: Trans-Exclusive Radical Feminist; originally referred to radical feminists who did not accept transgender ideology, but is currently used as a slur against anyone who does not fully capitulate to transgender activist's agenda.

Transgender: claiming to feel a mismatch between one's biological sex and one's sense of self; presenting oneself to the world according to stereotypes that do not align with those of one's biological (birth) sex.

Transphobia: fear or hatred of people who are transgender. In current vernacular this term is applied to anyone who disagrees with anything that a transgender person says, wants, or believes.

Unsupportive: unwilling to capitulate to all demands of the transgender-identified person.

Index

ENDNOTES

[1] Human Systems: Therapy, Culture and Attachment, Australian children and adolescents with gender dysphoria: Clinical presentations and challenges experienced by a multidisciplinary team and gender service. Kasia Kozlowska et al: https://journals.sagepub.com/doi/full/10.1177/26344041211010777

[2] Diagnostic and Statistical Manual of Mental Disorders 5. American Psychiatric Association. 2013, p. 454. ISBN 978-0-89042-555-8.

[3] Standards of Care for the Health of Transsexual, Transgender, and GenderNonconforming People, The World Professional Association for Transgender Health: https://www.wpath.org/media/cms/Documents/SOC%20v7/SOC%20V7_English2012.pdf?_t=1613669341

[4] Zucker, K. J. (2019), Different strokes for different folks: Child and Adolescent Mental Health Journal.

[5] https://youtu.be/Vr8rz8THpk0

[6] Shrier, Abigail. *Irreversible Damage.* Salem Media Group, 2020.

[7] Doctor fired from gender identity clinic says he feels "vindicated" after CAMH apology, settlement, Molly Hayes. https://www.theglobeandmail.com/canada/toronto/article-doctor-fired-from-gender-identity-clinic-says-he-feels-vindicated/

[8] Tavistock trust whistleblower David Bell: "I believed I was doing the right thing," May 5, 2021, Rachel Cooke: https://www.theguardian.com/society/2021/may/02/tavistock-trust-whistleblower-david-bell-transgender-children-gids?fbclid=IwAR0kY95OrJ6dIC9_v2e11N2PPDE0jOtNv46kCcTR5GLHyFjT68a_fOqWqE0

[9] Wikipedia, Gender April, 2021: https://en.wikipedia.org/wiki/Gender

[10] https://www.hrc.org/resources/sexual-orientation-and-gender-identity-terminology-and-definitions

[11] https://www.aclupa.org/en/news/trans-women-are-women-avoiding-mistakes-our-predecessors

[12] Bret Weinstein and Heather Heying - Gender Ideology vs Biology: https://www.youtube.com/watch?v=7xU77FhkcZ8

[13] Biological Theories of Gender, Dr. Saul McLeod:

https://www.simplypsychology.org/gender-biology.html

[14] Gender Ideology in Our Schools: https://youtu.be/KkmmEHvlpTk

[15] Genders Spectrum, April, 2021: https://www.genderspectrum.org/

[16] [Tailer] Not My Cup Of T (prior to release of "Dyshporic") by Vaishnavi Sundar, Sasha Ayad: https://www.youtube.com/playlist?list=PLRU9NIX0AA143z2QKukQcOqS96qriKGyw

[17] The Mayo Clinic, dissociative disorders: https://www.mayoclinic.org/diseases-conditions/dissociative-disorders/symptoms-causes/syc-20355215#:~:text=Dissociative%20disorders%20are%20mental%20disorders,with%20functioning%20in%20everyday%20life

[18] Human Rights Campaign, Transgender Children & Youth: Understanding the Basics: https://www.hrc.org/resources/transgender-children-and-youth-understanding-the-basics

[19] Orwell, George, and Erich Fromm. 1984. New York, NY: New American Library, 1961.

[20] Diagnostic and Statistical Manual of Mental Disorders 5. American Psychiatric Association, 2013, p. 454. ISBN 978-0-89042-555-8.

[21] Zucker, K. J. (2019). Different strokes for different folks. Child and Adolescent Mental Health Journal.

[22] Doctor fired from gender identity clinic says he feels "vindicated" after CAMH apology, settlement, Molly Hayes.

[23] https://www.mayoclinic.org/diseases-conditions/gender-dysphoria/symptoms-causes/syc-20475255

[24] Exploring the Domestic Abuse Narratives of Trans and Nonbinary People and the Role of Cisgenderism in Identity Abuse, Misgendering, and Pathologizing Michaela M. Rogers: https://journals.sagepub.com/doi/full/10.1177/1077801220971368

[25] Transgender Health Survey https://transequality.org/issues/us-trans-survey

[26] https://youtu.be/2iJHf1BKPJY

[27] https://segm.org/

[28] https://journals.sagepub.com/doi/full/10.1177/26344041211010777

[29] Childhood Sexual Abuse, Gender Dysphoria, and Transition Regret: Billy's Story, Walt Heyer: https://www.thepublicdiscourse.com/2018/03/21178/

[30] Responding to Transgender Victims of Sexual Assault: https://ovc.ojp.gov/sites/g/files/xyckuh226/files/pubs/forge/sexual_ch_e.html

[31] Female detransition and reidentification: Survey results and interpretation https://guideonragingstars.tumblr.com/post/149877706175/female-detransition-and-reidentification-survey

[32] Why I Transitioned & Detransitioned, Elle Palmer: https://youtu.be/n0pVuZ0CT7Q

[33] 12 Causes of Gender Dysphoria: Melinda Selmys: https://www.patheos.com/blogs/catholicauthenticity/2015/07/12-causes-of-gender-dysphoria/

[34] Tavistock trust whistleblower David Bell: "I believed I was doing the right thing," May 5, 2021, Rachel Cooke: https://www.theguardian.com/society/2021/may/02/tavistock-trust-whistleblower-david-bell-transgender-children-gids?fbclid=IwAR0kY95OrJ6dIC9_v2e11N2PPDE0jOtNv46kCcTR5GLHyFjT68a_fOqWqE0

[35] Understanding Gender Nonconformity, Dr. Robert Garofalo: https://youtu.be/zcJYq9U3v74

[36] Autism and Gender Identity, Nem: https://youtu.be/GjXcK77XjdY

[37] Testosterone, Mastectomy, Hysterectomy, Then Detransition, Ashira: https://youtu.be/i0EFPv1_jdI

[38] Data & Statistics on Autism Spectrum Disorder: https://www.cdc.gov/ncbddd/autism/data.html

[39] Human Systems: Therapy, Culture and Attachment, Australian children and adolescents with gender dysphoria: Clinical presentations and challenges experienced by a multidisciplinary team and gender service, Kasia Kozlowska et al: https://journals.sagepub.com/doi/full/10.1177/26344041211010777

[40] National Outcome Measure 17.3: Percent of children, ages 3 through 17, diagnosed with an autism spectrum disorder: https://www.childhealthdata.org/browse/survey/results?q=5425&r=1&gclid=Cj0KCQjw1a6EBhC0ARIsAOiTkrGYLr8KHA_dKUnCLx-TJPA67gEwYOZh4gR1gO_rO7twaFQgKlPxBsYaAkFaEALw_wcB

[41] Wishing to be another gender: Links to ADHD, autism spectrum disorders: https://www.sciencedaily.com/releases/2014/03/140312103102.htm

[42] https://guideonragingstars.tumblr.com/post/149877706175/female-detransition-and-reidentification-survey

[43] Largest study to date confirms overlap between autism and gender diversity, Laura Dattaro: https://www.spectrumnews.org/news/largest-study-to-date-confirms-overlap-between-autism-and-gender-diversity/

[44] Outbreak: On Transgender Teens and Psychic Epidemics, Lisa Marchiano: https://www.tandfonline.com/doi/full/10.1080/00332925.2017.1350804

[45] Parent reports of adolescents and young adults perceived to show signs of a rapid onset of gender dysphoria, Lisa Littman: https://journals.plos.org/plosone/article?id=10.1371/journal.pone.0202330

[46] Female detransition and reidentification: Survey results and interpretation https://guideonragingstars.tumblr.com/post/149877706175/female-detransition-and-reidentification-survey

[47] Shrier, A. (2020). *Irreversible Damage: The Transgender Craze Seducing Our Daughters.*

[48] 11th Hour Blog, Follow the Money: How the Pritzker Family Makes a Killing From the Transgender Industry, Jennifer Bilek: https://www.the11thhourblog.com/

[49] Menno, Gays Against Gender (G.A.G.) Part 1-3: https://youtu.be/q13Cju4IhV8

[50] Andrea O'Brien, personal communication.

[51] Diagnostic and Statistical Manual of Mental Disorders 5. American Psychiatric Association. 2013. ISBN 978-0-89042-555-8.

[52] Report: Gay Iranians Coerced Into Gender Reassignment Surgery: Homosexuals in the Islamic Republic are being pressured into changing their gender in order to "fix" them, the BBC reports: https://www.haaretz.com/gays-in-iran-pressured-to-change-gender-1.5325533

[53] Trans-Identity Development: Potential Causes, Sydney Wright: https://vimeo.com/manage/videos/490953579

[54] Sex, Lies, and Children Protecting the Vulnerable from Irreversible Harm, Sydney Wright Testimony for Alabama VCAP legislation.

[55] Children's Rights, Trans Realities, Scott Newgent: https://youtu.be/Lly1prUzksI

[56] Kai Shappley: A Trans Girl Growing Up In Texas, Emmy-Winning Documentary: https://www.youtube.com/watch?v=cuIkLNsRtas

[57] Transgender Kids: Who Knows Best. BBC: https://www.bbc.co.uk/programmes/b088kxbw

[58] TEDxTWU Transgender kids are just kids after all, Amber Briggle: https://www.youtube.com/watch?v=t_gCASi58Ps&t=

[59] NHS child gender clinic: Staff welfare concerns "shut down." BBC Newsnight, Debrah Cohen: https://youtu.be/zTRnrp9pXHY

[60] Rep. Marie Newman Absurd Claims in Defense of Equality Act: https://youtu.be/XNrNY31Qzcs

[61] https://youtu.be/zTRnrp9pXHY

[62] Lisa Wilson, Personal Communication

[63] MTF Detransition, Josh Drewes, https://youtu.be/ivqdxLUbq3Q

[64] MtFtM Detransition 5, Kevin, Q&A: https://youtu.be/0ULb3kG_21c

[65] Michael Bailey. 2003. *The Man Who Would Be Queen: The Science of Gender-Bending and Transsexualism.* Washington, DC: Joseph Henry Press.

[66] MtFtM Detransition 5, Kevin, Q&A: https://youtu.be/0ULb3kG_21c

[67] A History of Autogynephilia, Maranda Yardly: https://mirandayardley.com/en/a-history-of-autogynephilia/

[68] Gender Colonialism, Nina Paley: https://blog.ninapaley.com/2018/02/07/gender_colonialism/

[69] TRA violent threats: https://photos.google.com/share/AF1QipOM9J_ZIrYtiMagVRr_jhagMR-XP59TBsJFLwNlcS13iIUT4ovqKRN9zttevr0PmA?pli=1&fbclid=IwAR0wDBFMLOc-XS1ffVH4HTeYyD9yJ7lQdxo8v3kxOdtgDrz0mIeXZuwH0ak&key=NmJuV1AyRnVSU3dOS2VObVhLSm1uNUkxRjRBSk9R

[70] https://www.reddit.com/r/sissyhypno/

[71] https://grahamlinehan.substack.com/p/sissy-porn-the-gender-movements-dirty

[72] https://www.versobooks.com/books/3061-females

[73] https://www.hhs.gov/answers/mental-health-and-substance-abuse/what-does-suicide-contagion-mean/index.html#:~:text=Suicide%20contagion%20is%20the%20exposure,in%20suicide%20and%20suicidal%20behaviors

[74] Dr. Kevin Stuart's Testimony on SB 131: https://youtu.be/zhRW02Sn3Nw

[75] Puberty blockers: Under-16s "unlikely" to be able to give informed consent, BBC Newsnight Susie green, the CEO of mermaid to charity, https://youtu.be/0A6dFxAf8wY

[76] An Evening With Dr Stanley Biber 1997, Dr. Stanley Biber: https://youtu.be/R4b4U9zjlsk

[77] Gender Dysphoria Treatment, Dr. Norman Spack: https://youtu.be/0tqil7Audws

[78] https://www.aclu.org/news/lgbtq-rights/doctors-agree-gender-affirming-care-is-life-saving-care/

[79] How Trans Kids And Their Parents Decide When To Start Medical Transition, Dr. Elizabeth Miller: https://youtu.be/QD720mHFqW0

[80] https://www.advocate.com/commentary/2021/5/03/im-doctor-gender-affirming-care-saves-trans-lives

[81] https://www.cnn.com/2020/01/23/health/transgender-puberty-blockers-suicide-study/index.html

[82] https://fearlessbr.com/lgbtq-gender-affirming-care-guest-opinion/

[83] HB1057 Senate Committee Hearing: Vulnerable Child Protection Act, Dr. Keith Hansen: https://youtu.be/AHDpZ7SIr78

[84] The Tavistock's Experiment with Puberty Blockers* Michael Biggs Department of Sociology and St Cross College, University of Oxford (version 1.0.1, 29 July 2019): http://users.ox.ac.uk/~sfos0060/Biggs_ExperimentPubertyBlockers.pdf

[85] Correction to Bränström and Pachankis. Published Online:1 Aug 2020 https://doi.org/10.1176/appi.ajp.2020.1778 correction https://ajp.psychiatryonline.org/doi/10.1176/appi.ajp.2020.1778correction

[86] Sweden's Karolinska Ends All Use of Puberty Blockers and Cross-Sex Hormones for Minors Outside of Clinical Studies, https://segm.org/Sweden_ends_use_of_Dutch_protocol

[87] Puberty blockers: "We need facts and evidence, not ideology," Bev Jackson: https://youtu.be/OEAkU0asJZg

[88] Pennsylvania State House, Dr. Stephen Levine: https://www.tandfonline.com/doi/full/10.1080/0092623X.2017.1309482?scrol l=top&needAccess=true

[89] VCAP Hearings, Alabama 2020, Dr. Patrick Lappert.

[90] Wallace Wong, 27 Feb. 2019: https://vimeo.com/326339802

[91] Transgender Surgery Provides No Mental Health Benefit, Dr. Andre Van Mol, https://youtu.be/f4cX1ZdE8PY

[92] Pediatric Endocrinologist Fights Against Harmful Trans Ideology, Dr. Quentin Van Meter: https://youtu.be/lcYrDrzV7DY

[93] Pediatric Endocrinologist Fights Against Harmful Trans Ideology, Dr. Quentin Van Meter: https://youtu.be/lcYrDrzV7DY

[94] Transforming Gender (Transgender Documentary), Olie's Father: https://youtu.be/B67OVJTyV0I

[95] How Trans Kids And Their Parents Decide When To Start Medical Transition, Max's Mother: https://youtu.be/QD720mHFqW0

[96] National Center for Transgender Equality US Transgender Survey, 2015: https://www.ustranssurvey.org/

[97] How Trans Kids And Their Parents Decide When To Start Medical Transition, Kimberly Shapley: https://youtu.be/QD720mHFqW0

[98] Injustice at Every Turn: A Report of the National Transgender Discrimination Survey https://transequality.org/sites/default/files/docs/resources/NTDS_Report.pd f

[99] The Keira Bell Case and A New Therapeutic Model, Marcus Evans: https://youtu.be/HC3KzgtEW08

[100] Transgender Kids Who Knows Best, Lou: https://www.bbc.co.uk/programmes/b088kxbw

[101] House Health and Human Services Policy Committee, part 1 2/13/19, Luca Groppoli: https://youtu.be/2NEK9M-FjIs

[102] Transgender Moment Conference: Panel on Medicine, Dr. Paul Hruz: https://youtu.be/bhHjsvr1AcM

[103] Vulnerable Child Protection Legislation: Texas Hearings Senate Bills 1311 and 64: https://youtu.be/RxAtDk5wXh4

[104] The Role of Behavioral Health in Gender Affirming Care, UCLA MDChat, Dr. Brandon Ito: https://youtu.be/XZR5OFfdEWI

[105] The Hormone Health Crisis with Endocrinologist William Malone, MD, Dr. William Malone: https://youtu.be/z4RYl75zdMY

[106] Recommendations for Reporting on Suicide: https://www.datocms-assets.com/12810/1577098761-recommendations.pdf

[107] Public Discourse, The Pediatric Endocrine Society's Statement on Puberty Blockers Isn't Just Deceptive. It's Dangerous. Dr. Michael Laidlaw: https://www.thepublicdiscourse.com/2020/01/59422/

[108] The terrible fraud of transgender medicine, Quentin Van Meter: https://youtu.be/6mtQ1geeD_c

[109] Harry Benjamin's first ten cases (1938–1953): a clinical historical note. Arch Sex Behav, Schaefer LC, Wheeler CC. 1995; 24(1):73–93. doi:10.1007/BF01541990.

[110] John Money, David Reimer, and the Dark Origins of the Transgender Movement, George Luke: https://www.intellectualtakeout.org/article/john-money-david-reimer-and-dark-origins-transgender-movement/

[111] Johns Hopkins psychiatrist sees hospital come full circle on transgender issues Amy Ellis Nutt, The Washington Post, April 06, 2017: https://www.baltimoresun.com/health/bal-johns-hopkins-transgender-20170406-story.html

[112] Lupron Victims Hub: https://www.lupronvictimshub.com/lawsuits.html

[113] Testosterone Lawsuits: https://www.drugwatch.com/testosterone/lawsuits/#:~:text=Many%20lawsuits%20name%20Abbvie's%20testosterone,not%20disclose%20the%20settlement%20amount

[114] Using HRT (Hormone Replacement Therapy): https://www.breastcancer.org/risk/factors/hrt

[115] Christina Jewett, "Women Fear Drug They Used To Halt Puberty Led To Health

Problems," Kaiser Health News (February 2, 2017): https://khn.org/news/women-fear-drug-they-used-to-halt-puberty- led-to-health-problems/

[116] Maiko A Schneider, et al., "Brain Maturation, Cognition and Voice Pattern in a Gender Dysphoria articles/10.3389/fnhum.2017.00528/full; Peter Hayes, "Commentary: Cognitive, Emotional, and Psychosocial Functioning of Girls Treated with Pharmacological Puberty Blockage for Idiopathic Central Precocious Puberty" Frontiers in Psychology 8(44) (February 2017), https://www.ncbi.nlm.nih.gov/pmc/articles/PMC5253377/#!po=10.0000

[117] Hruz, et al., "Growing Pains: Problems with Puberty Suppression," supra n. 10.

[118] Norman P. Spack, et al., "Children and Adolescents With Gender Identity Disorder Referred to a Pediatric Medical Center" Pediatrics 129(3):418–425 (March 12), https://pediatrics.aappublications. org/content/129/3/418; Michael Laidlaw, Michelle Cretella, Kevin Donovan, The Right to Best Care for Children Does Not Include the Right to Medical Transition, American Journal of Bioethics, 19 (2):75–77 (2019). https://doi.org/10.1080/15265161.2018.1557288

[119] Combaz N, Kuhn A, "Long-Term Urogynecological Complications after Sex Reassignment Surgery in Transsexual Patients: a Retrospective Study of 44 Patients and Diagnostic Algorithm Proposal," Am J Urol Res. 2017; 2(2): 038–043. https://www.scireslit.com/Urology/AJUR-ID21.pdf, Rossi Neto, R., et. al., "Gender reassignment surgery - a 13 year review of surgical outcomes" International Braz J. Urol., 38(1), 97-107 (2012) https://dx.doi.org/10.1590/S1677-55382012000100014

[120] Dr. Johanna Olson-Kennedy explains why mastectomies for healthy teen girls is no big deal: https://youtu.be/5Y6espcXPJk

[121] Kaiser-Permanente: Mastectomy for healthy 12 (TWELVE) year old girl, Kellyn Lakhardt of Kaiser Permanente: https://youtu.be/E38o16gyBuI

[122] Society for Evidence Based Gender Medicine: https://segm.org/

[123] Utah Sees 10,000% Increase in Girls Getting "Sex Change," Alex Newman: https://thenewamerican.com/utah-sees-10-000-increase-in-girls-getting-sex-change/

[124] How to tell if babies are transgender? Diane Ehrensaft: https://youtu.be/M7KBZeRC1RI

[125] Eight Year Olds Are Being Given Cross-Gender Hormones, Erin Brewer: https://www.chooseyourowndiagnosis.com/2019/03/eight-year-olds-are-being-given-cross.html

[126] How Cognitive Behavioral Therapy Can Rewire Your Thoughts: https://www.healthline.com/health/cognitive-behavioral-therapy

[127] The DSM-5 and the Politics of Diagnosing Transpeople. Davy Z. Arch Sex Behav.

2015 Jul; 44(5):1165–76. doi: 10.1007/s10508-015-0573-6. PMID: 26054486.

[128] Diagnostic and Statistical Manual of Mental Disorders 5. American Psychiatric Association. 2013. p. 454. ISBN 978-0-89042-555-8.

[129] Report of the APA Task Force on Treatment of Gender Identity Disorder, William Byne MD, PhD, Am J Psychiatry 169:8, August 2012, data supplement.

[130] WPATH. (2012). *Standards of Care version 7*. WPATH Standards of Care. https://wpath.org/publications/soc

[131] French, Helen 3, 8, 2018 Clinical Leader: Legal & Ethical Considerations For Informed Consent In Clinical Trials https://www.clinicalleader.com/doc/legal-ethical-considerations-for-informed-consent-in-clinical-trials-0001

[132] Understanding Transgender Issues: An Interview with Dr. Patrick Lappert, Family Watch International, Dr. Patrick Lappert: https://vimeo.com/498679928

[133] Richard Bränström, John E. Pachankis, Reduction in Mental Health Treatment Utilization Among Transgender Individuals After Gender-Affirming Surgeries: A Total Population Study: http://ajp.psychiatryonline.org/doi/full/10.1176/appi.ajp.2019.19010080

[134] Long-Term Follow-Up of Transsexual Persons Undergoing Sex Reassignment Surgery: Cohort Study in Sweden Cecilia Dhejne, Paul Lichtenstein, Marcus Boman, Anna L. V. Johansson, Niklas Långström, Mikael Landén: https://journals.plos.org/plosone/article?id=10.1371/journal.pone.0016885#:~:text=Our%20findings%20suggest%20that%20sex,reassignment%20for%20this%20is%20patient%20group

[135] Long-Term Follow-Up of Transsexual Persons Undergoing Sex Reassignment Surgery: Cohort Study in Sweden Cecilia Dhejne, Paul Lichtenstein, Marcus Boman, Anna L. V. Johansson, Niklas Långström, Mikael Landén: https://journals.plos.org/plosone/article?id=10.1371/journal.pone.0016885#:~:text=Our%20findings%20suggest%20that%20sex,reassignment%20for%20this%20is%20patient%20group

[136] Parent reports of adolescents and young adults perceived to show signs of a rapid onset of gender dysphoria, Lisa Littman: https://journals.plos.org/plosone/article?id=10.1371/journal.pone.0202330

[137] Safeguarding adolescents from premature, permanent medicalization, Susan Bewley: https://www.bmj.com/content/364/bmj.l245/rr-1

[138] Tavistock clinic reveals surge in girls switching gender, Andrew Gilligan: https://www.thetimes.co.uk/article/surge-in-girls-switching-gender-pwqdtd5vk

[139] Tavistock trust whistleblower David Bell: "I believed I was doing the right thing," May 5, 2021, 9 Rachel Cooke: https://www.theguardian.com/society/2021/may/02/tavistock-trust-whistleblower-david-bell-transgender-children-gids?fbclid=IwAR0kY95OrJ6dIC9_v2e11N2PPDE0jOtNv46kCcTR5GLHyFj

T68a_fOqWqE0

[140] Bell v Tavistock Judgement: https://www.judiciary.uk/wp-content/uploads/2020/12/Bell-v-Tavistock-Judgment.pdf

[141] The Rise of Transgender Medicine, https://www.youtube.com/watch?v=OGbz57wZ28A&t=11s

[142] Affirmative Quackery: Harry Benjamin and WPATH https://stoptransingkids.wordpress.com/2020/06/02/who-was-harry-benjamin/

[143] Standards of Care for the Health of Transsexual, Transgender, and GenderNonconforming People, The World Professional Association for Transgender Health: https://www.wpath.org/media/cms/Documents/SOC%20v7/SOC%20V7_English2012.pdf?_t=1613669341

[144] Gender identity clinic accused of fast-tracking young adults, Jamie Doward: https://www.theguardian.com/society/2018/nov/03/tavistock-centre-gender-identity-clinic-accused-fast-tracking-young-adults

[145] Eight Year Olds Are Being Given Cross-Gender Hormones, Erin Brewer: https://www.chooseyourowndiagnosis.com/2019/03/eight-year-olds-are-being-given-cross.html

[146] Dr. Johanna Olson-Kennedy explains why mastectomies for healthy teen girls are no big deal: https://youtu.be/5Y6espcXPJk

[147] Dahlen S, Connolly D, Arif I, et al, International clinical practice guidelines for gender minority/trans people: systematic review and quality assessment BMJ Open 2021; 11:e048943. doi: 10.1136/bmjopen-2021-048943: https://t.co/3XM1z91a9p?amp=1

[148] Understanding Transgender Issues: Interview with Dr. Michelle Cretella, Family Watch International, Dr. Michelle Cretella: https://vimeo.com/498975226

[149] Equality Utah letter regarding conversion therapy ban, personal communication 2019.

[150] Woman treated with hormone blockers to reassign gender takes NHS to court: https://youtu.be/BKVSr7OMetU

[151] I Regret Top Surgery: https://youtu.be/1s1dMKk_CK4

[152] "Understanding Gender Nonconformity in Children and Adolescents" by Dr. Robert Garofalo https://youtu.be/zcJYq9U3v74

[153] Female detransition and reidentification: Survey results and interpretation https://guideonragingstars.tumblr.com/post/149877706175/female-detransition-and-reidentification-survey

[154] Tavistock trust whistleblower David Bell: 'I believed I was doing the right thing'

May 5, 2021, Rachel Cooke:
https://www.theguardian.com/society/2021/may/02/tavistock-trust-whistleblower-david-bell-transgender-children-gids

[155] Human Systems: Therapy, Culture and Attachment, Australian children and adolescents with gender dysphoria: Clinical presentations and challenges experienced by a multidisciplinary team and gender service, Kasia Kozlowska et al: https://journals.sagepub.com/doi/full/10.1177/26344041211010777

[156] Decision-Making Is Still A Work In Progress For Teenagers: https://brainconnection.brainhq.com/2013/03/20/decision-making-is-still-a-work-in-progress-for-teenagers/

[157] The New Atlantis, Growing Pains: Problems with Puberty Suppression in Treating Gender Dysphoria, Paul Hruz, Lawrence Mayer, Paul McHugh: https://www.thenewatlantis.com/publications/growing-pains

[158] "Looking at suppressing puberty for transgender kids." Associated Press. March 12, 2016.

[159] "Transgender Youth Using Puberty Blockers." KQED. August 19, 2016.

[160] Alegría, Christine Aramburu (2016-10-01). "Gender nonconforming and transgender children/youth: Family, community, and implications for practice." Journal of the American Association of Nurse Practitioners. 28 (10): 521–527. doi:10.1002/2327-6924.12363. ISSN 2327-6924. PMID 27031444.

[161] Current treatments for endometriosis, Mayo Clininc, https://www.mayoclinic.org/diseases-conditions/endometriosis/diagnosis-treatment/drc-20354661

[162] More women come forward with complaints about Lupron side effects: https://www.ktnv.com/news/investigations/more-women-come-forward-with-complaints-about-lupron-side-effects

[163] Mom celebrates her teen's puberty-blocker induced early menopause. A mom took to the internet to croon with pride for her 15-year-old child who is undergoing early, medically induced, menopause, Libby Emmons Brooklyn, NY, 19th April 2020.

[164] Klink D, Caris M, Heijboer A, van Trotsenburg M, Rotteveel J, Bone Mass in Young Adulthood Following Gonadotropin-Releasing Hormone Analog Treatment and Cross-Sex Hormone Treatment in Adolescents With Gender Dysphoria, J. CLINICAL ENDO. & MET AB., Vol.I 00(2) E270-E275 (I Feb 2015) https://doi.org/ I 0.121O/jc.2014-2439

[165] The Tavistock's Experiment with Puberty Blockers* Michael Biggs Department of Sociology and St Cross College, University of Oxford (version 1.0.1, 29 July 2019): http://users.ox.ac.uk/~sfos0060/Biggs_ExperimentPubertyBlockers.pdf

[166] Women fear drug they used to halt puberty led to health problems, Darcy Spears: https://www.pbs.org/newshour/health/women-fear-drug-they-used-to-halt-

puberty-led-to-health-problems

[167] Lupron Victim Advocate Issues Urgent Warning, November 11, 2019: https://www.kelseycoalition.org/pubs/Lupron-Victim-Advocate-Issues-Urgent-Warning

[168] Transgender Surgery Provides No Mental Health Benefit, Andre Van Mol: https://www.youtube.com/watch?v=f4cX1ZdE8PY&t=802s

[169] Veteran Plastic Surgeon: No One Is Born In The Wrong Body, Dr. Patrick Lappert: https://youtu.be/wtG7rJdxAZg

[170] Pediatric Endocrinologist Fights Against Harmful Trans Ideology, Dr. Quentin Van Meter, https://youtu.be/lcYrDrzV7DY

[171] Pennsylvania Public Hearing on Appropriate Care Models for Transgender Adolescents, Dr. Stephen Levine: http://www.pahousegop.com/embed/24641/Public-hearing-on-Appropriate-Care-Models-for-Transgender-Adolescents-

[172] The Impact of Early Medical Treatments in Transgender Youth, Johanna Olson: https://docs.wixstatic.com/ugd/3f4f51_a929d049f7fb46c7a72c4c86ba43869a.pdf

[173] Buck Angel interview with Scarlet. https://www.instagram.com/p/CN8DVvVjbKR/

[174] Dr. Johanna Olson-Kennedy explains why mastectomies for healthy teen girls is no big deal: https://youtu.be/5Y6espcXPJk

[175] Kaiser-Permanente: Mastectomy for healthy 12 (TWELVE) year old girl Kellyn Lakhardt of the Kaiser Permanente: https://youtu.be/E38o16gyBuI

[176] https://www.plannedparenthood.org/learn/teens/ask-experts/i-have-been-with-my-girlfriend-for-just-over-two-years-we-have-been-having-sex-for-a-rather-long-time-we-have-tried-a-variety-of-different-contraceptives-but-after-a-rather-lengthy-conversation-wit

[177] Stella O'Malley on Detransition Conference and medical ethics in the age of gender identity, Stella O'Malley, https://youtu.be/G5G-Jg6prkc

[178] House Health and Human Services Committee - February 19, 2021 hearing, Dr. Nicole Mihalopoulos: https://le.utah.gov/av/committeeArchive.jsp?timelineID=180777

[179] Detransition-Related Needs and Support: A Cross-Sectional Online Survey Elie Vandenbussche: https://www.tandfonline.com/doi/full/10.1080/00918369.2021.1919479?fbclid=IwAR2ULGen9ncdud-X1QxFq_5ZyC57Z9P3j4u-f4SRIEfpvqTYonGoA8qGE90.

[180] MTF Detransition, Josh Drewes, https://youtu.be/ivqdxLUbq3Q

181 Detransitioning is Not Taboo, Waffling Willow: https://youtu.be/d-z4H4NvGjw

182 HB1057 Senate Committee Hearing - Vulnerable Child Protection Act, Statement by Sydney Wright: https://youtu.be/AHDpZ7SIr78

183 [Trailer] Not My Cup Of T (prior to release of "Dyshporic") by Vaishnavi Sundar, Sasha Ayad: https://www.youtube.com/playlist?list=PLRU9NIX0AA143z2QKukQcOqS96qriKGyw

184 MtFtM Detransition 5 – Kevin: Q&A https://youtu.be/0ULb3kG_21c

185 My experience with Planned Parenthood, Rival Maverick: https://youtu.be/TMOKaZd7OFE

186 My reasons for detransitioning (ftm detransition), Leoaica Motanelul: https://www.youtube.com/watch?v=lsnV5heKerc

187 His Body Wasn't Wrong, His Thoughts Were, Billy Burleigh: https://youtu.be/55IR8taw2Ig

188 #2 James Caspian: Censoring studies on trans people: https://youtu.be/t_7BMRqPtWs

189 Billy's Story: https://vimeo.com/525686944

190 Testosterone, Mastectomy, Hysterectomy, Then Detransition, Ashira: https://youtu.be/i0EFPv1_jdI

191 Transgender Surgery: "What Have I Done?" Leoaica Motanelul: https://vimeo.com/500280130

192 House Health and Human Services Committee - February 19, 2021 hearing, Dr. Nicole Mihalopoulos: https://le.utah.gov/av/committeeArchive.jsp?timelineID=180777

193 When Children Say They're Trans, Jesse Singal: https://www.theatlantic.com/magazine/archive/2018/07/when-a-child-says-shes-trans/561749/

194 Prismic. (n.d.). *Gender Spectrum HomepageGender Spectrum*. Gender Spectrum. http://genderspectrum.org/

195 *What Schools Are Doing*. Arlington Parent Coalition. (n.d.). https://arlingtonparentcoa.wixsite.com/arlingtonparentcoa/what-schools-are-doing.

196 GLSEN. (n.d.). *GLSEN Model School District Policy*. www.glsen.org. https://www.glsen.org/sites/default/files/2019-10/GLSEN-Model-School-District-Policy-Transgender-Gender-Nonconforming-Students.pdf.

197 *Do You Know What Your Kids Are Reading at School?* Arlington Parent Coalition. (2020, April 21). https://arlingtonparentcoa.wixsite.com/arlingtonparentcoa/post/do-you-

know-what-your-kids-are-reading-at-school.

[198] Planned Parenthood (n.d.). *Sex Education Tools for Educators: Sex Education Resources.* Planned Parenthood. https://www.plannedparenthood.org/learn/for-educators.

[199] Keffler, M. (2020, December 7). *Peer-Led Sex Ed: Marketing Gender to Kids at School.* Partners for Ethical Care. https://www.partnersforethicalcare.com/post/peer-led-sex-ed-marketing-gender-to-kids-at-school.

[200] Yahoo! (n.d.). *school+posters+LGBTQ.* Yahoo! https://images.search.yahoo.com/search/images;_ylt=A0geKeQoccRgmw0Aj8tXNyoA;_ylu=Y29sbwNiZjEEcG9zAzEEdnRpZAMEc2VjA3BpdnM-?p=school%2Bposters%2BLGBTQ&fr2=piv-web&fr=mcafee.

[201] *Gender ID Indoctrination for 4th & 5th Graders at Oakridge.* Arlington Parent Coalition. (2020, January 9). https://arlingtonparentcoa.wixsite.com/arlingtonparentcoa/post/gender-id-indoctrination-for-4th-5th-graders-at-oakridge.

[202] *Here's Exactly Why the APS Default Sex-Ed Opt-Out Form Is Useless.* Arlington Parent Coalition. (2019, September 28). https://arlingtonparentcoa.wixsite.com/arlingtonparentcoa/post/here-s-exactly-why-the-aps-default-sex-ed-opt-out-form-is-useless.

[203] *GSA Mission Statement Examples.* American Civil Liberties Union. (n.d.). https://www.aclu.org/other/gsa-mission-statement-examples.

[204] Keffler, M. (2021, February 8). *Horrified Mother Gets Front Row Seat to Sex & Gender Indoctrination Strategy Meeting.* Partners for Ethical Care. https://www.partnersforethicalcare.com/post/horrified-mother-gets-front-row-seat-to-sex-gender-indoctrination-strategy-meeting.

[205] Truong, D. (2019, March 3). *In a Virginia school, a celebration of transgender students in a kindergarten class.* The Washington Post. https://www.washingtonpost.com/local/education/in-a-virginia-school-a-celebration-of-transgender-students-in-a-kindergarten-class/2019/03/03/10fc9f90-3b7e-11e9-a06c-3ec8ed509d15_story.html.

[206] *Not In Favor Of Your Kids Celebrating Sex at School? You Might Want to Be Aware...* Arlington Parent Coalition. (2019, November 12). https://arlingtonparentcoa.wixsite.com/arlingtonparentcoa/post/not-in-favor-of-your-kids-celebrating-sex-at-school-you-might-want-to-be-aware.

[207] *Counselor Using Naviance to Distribute LGB/TQ Activism Advertisements.* Arlington Parent Coalition. (2020, March 12). https://arlingtonparentcoa.wixsite.com/arlingtonparentcoa/post/counselor-using-naviance-to-distribute-lgb-tq-activism-advertisements.

[208] Keffler, M. (2020, December 23). *Transgender Religion Codified & Enforced at School.* Partners for Ethical Care.

https://www.partnersforethicalcare.com/post/transgender-religion-codified-enforced-at-school.

[209] Alliance Defending Freedom. (2019, September 30). *The Peter Vlaming Case.* Vlaming v. West Point School Board. https://adflegal.org/sites/default/files/2020-09/Vlaming%20v.%20West%20Point%20School%20Board%20-%20One-page%20summary.pdf.

[210] Bilek, J. (2018, February 22). *Who Are the Rich, White Men Institutionalizing Transgender Ideology?* The Federalist. https://thefederalist.com/2018/02/20/rich-white-men-institutionalizing-transgender-ideology/.

[211] Keffler, M. (2021). *Desist, detrans & detox: getting your child out of the gender cult.* International Partners for Ethical Care.

[212] Chen, G. (2008, March 26). Parental Involvement is Key to Student Success. Retrieved August 19, 2020, from https://www.publicschoolreview.com/blog/parental-involvement-is-key-to-student-success.

[213] Gallagher, M., Dalrymple, T., Donald, H., & McGinnis, J. (2019, June 18). Why Marriage Is Good For You. Retrieved August 19, 2020, from https://www.city-journal.org/html/why-marriage-good-you-12002.html.

[214] Linehan, G. (2021, January 23). Another central OUTLIER: Rachel McKinnon. Retrieved February 16, 2021, from https://grahamlinehan.substack.com/p/another-central-outlier-rachel-mckinnon.

[215] National Society for the Prevention of Cruelty to Children. (n.d.). Grooming. Retrieved August 19, 2020, from https://www.nspcc.org.uk/what-is-child-abuse/types-of-abuse/grooming/.

[216] Gladwell, M. (2012, September 17). In Plain View. Retrieved August 19, 2020, from https://www.newyorker.com/magazine/2012/09/24/in-plain-view.

[217] Keffler, M. (2021, February 8). *Horrified Mother Gets Front Row Seat to Sex & Gender Indoctrination Strategy Meeting.* Partners for Ethical Care. https://www.partnersforethicalcare.com/post/horrified-mother-gets-front-row-seat-to-sex-gender-indoctrination-strategy-meeting.

[218] Newman, A. (2020, August 15). *Teacher Recruits "Most Emotionally Unstable" Kids for LGBT Club.* The New American. https://thenewamerican.com/teacher-recruits-most-emotionally-unstable-kids-for-lgbt-club/.

[219] GLSEN. (n.d.). *GLSEN Model School District Policy.* www.glsen.org. https://www.glsen.org/sites/default/files/2019-10/GLSEN-Model-School-District-Policy-Transgender-Gender-Nonconforming-Students.pdf.

[220] *Schools In Transition.* HRC. (n.d.). https://www.hrc.org/resources/schools-in-transition-a-guide-for-supporting-transgender-students-in-k-12-s.

[221] American School Counselor Association. (n.d.). *The School Counselor and Transgender/Gender-nonconforming Youth*. The School Counselor and Transgender/Gender-nonconforming Youth - American School Counselor Association (ASCA). https://www.schoolcounselor.org/Standards-Positions/Position-Statements/ASCA-Position-Statements/The-School-Counselor-and-Transgender-Gender-noncon.

[222] Keffler, M. (2020, December 23). *Transgender Religion Codified & Enforced at School*. Partners for Ethical Care. https://www.partnersforethicalcare.com/post/transgender-religion-codified-enforced-at-school.

[223] *National Association of Social Workers (NASW)*. NASW - National Associacion of Social Workers. (n.d.). https://www.socialworkers.org/about/ethics/code-of-ethics/code-of-ethics-english.

[224] Hecht, A. (2021, January 29). *The Secret Tactics of Glitter Moms: A Tale of Betrayal and Grooming*. The Gender Map. https://www.gendermapper.org/post/the-secret-tactics-of-glitter-moms-a-tale-of-betrayal-and-grooming.

[225] Christensen, J. (2018, February 17). *Judge gives grandparents custody of Ohio transgender teen*. CNN. https://www.cnn.com/2018/02/16/health/ohio-transgender-teen-hearing-judge-decision/index.html.

[226] Showalter, B. (2021, March 18). *Canadian father jailed after publicly objecting to minor daughter taking testosterone*. The Christian Post. https://www.christianpost.com/news/canadian-father-jailed-for-speaking-out-about-gender-transition.html.

[227] Keenan, J. (2019, April 3). *'Doctor' Advises Threatening Suicide To Get Trans Treatments For Kids*. The Federalist. https://thefederalist.com/2019/04/01/doctor-advises-threatening-suicide-get-transgender-treatments-kids/.

[228] Cooper, J. (2021, February 17). *The New Tuskegee Experiment: The Slow Death of Black Men by Transgenderism*. Partners for Ethical Care. https://www.partnersforethicalcare.com/post/the-new-tuskegee-experiment-the-slow-death-of-black-men-by-transgenderism.

[229] Dr. Andre Van Mol, Transgender Surgery Provides No Mental Health Benefit https://youtu.be/f4cX1ZdE8PY

Made in the USA
Columbia, SC
16 February 2025

53950577П00087